T0235210

# Healthcare and Artificial Intelligence

Bernard Nordlinger · Cédric Villani ·
Daniela Rus

Editors

# Healthcare and Artificial Intelligence

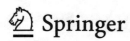 Springer

*Editors*
Bernard Nordlinger
Department of Surgery
Hôpital Ambroise Paré, Assistance
Publique Hôpitaux de Paris
Boulogne-Billancourt, France

Cédric Villani
Institut Henri Poincaré
Université de Lyon
Paris, France

Daniela Rus
Computer Science and Artificial Intelligence
Massachusetts Institute of Technology
Cambridge, MA, USA

ISBN 978-3-030-32163-5        ISBN 978-3-030-32161-1    (eBook)
https://doi.org/10.1007/978-3-030-32161-1

This Springer imprint is published by the registered company Springer Nature Switzerland AG
The registered company address is: Gewerbestrasse 11, 6330 Cham, Switzerland

# Foreword

This book is the result of a meeting between the mathematical Fields Medalist Cédric Villani, the brilliant surgeon Bernard Nordlinger, and the MacArthur Genius award-winning roboticist and computer scientist Daniela Rus. A priori, there was little to suggest they would ever work together: Cédric Villani was promoting mathematics as the head of the Raymond Poincaré Institute, Bernard Nordlinger was trying to improve the prognosis of cancers through ambitious therapeutic trials, and Daniela Rus was trying to create widely available robots and AI systems to support people with physical and cognitive work.

However, their meeting was not purely fortuitous since their trajectories crossed at an event in support of innovation and research. Bernard Nordlinger whose concerns extended beyond surgical procedure had extensive experience in controlled therapeutic trials. He was well aware of methodological requirements and the most appropriate means of exploiting the results. Cédric Villani whose interests went well beyond the world of mathematics was seeking advances that had the potential to be enabled across many fields (particularly, health). Daniela Rus was looking for advances having a societal impact (particularly, addressing significant challenges around curing disease).

Although their complementarity was obvious, it was necessary to provide a means of establishing exchanges between those who accumulated data and those who actively worked in particular fields. Cédric Villani and Bernard Nordlinger set up a joint working group between the French Academy of Sciences and the French Academy of Medicine. The working group comprised a number of highly qualified members of the two academies and many other experts. The objective of the working group was to meet to gather information, listen to presentations, and exchange ideas. Daniela Rus joined later and brought an American viewpoint and expertise.

A joint meeting of the two academies on "Mathematics, Big Data, and Health: The Example of Cancer" took place on November 28, 2017. By presenting examples from health insurance databases pertaining to results already obtained in imaging and genetics, they provided us with the first opportunity to highlight the prospects that mathematics could offer to the progress of science and technology in health.

The characteristics of health sciences and their "structural wounds" as Cédric Villani put it (more particularly, the complexity of phenomena, the variability of conclusions, the complexity of funding, and human interpretative bias) must find a new dynamic of progress by mobilizing mathematical sciences. By making it possible to exploit Big Data and, more generally, artificial intelligence, medicine will increase its means of action. No field of activity will be able to escape this evolution. The very special resonance that artificial intelligence will have in the health field should be obvious to all.

Renewing and perfecting the interpretation of images; increasing performance in radiology, pathological anatomy, and dermatology; taking advantage of genetic data; and developing precision medicine all will become possible thanks to artificial intelligence. It will enable the collection of data of a previously inaccessible richness to make possible the most careful clinical examinations. It will make an irreplaceable contribution to diagnostic and therapeutic choices.

Such a development presupposes the retraining of doctors and, more broadly, of health professionals. Such a change in practices also requires consideration of the evolution of responsibilities and their legal consequences. If the robot and the algorithm acquire such a critical role in the decision, will they assume a legal personality? The hopes raised by artificial intelligence raise questions and even concerns. These concerns are justified. The basic precaution is to be careful as we move toward the fantastic predictions of the "augmented man" that on the basis of adventurous extrapolations suggest a totally uncontrolled evolution.

We must thank Bernard Nordlinger, Cédric Villani, and Daniela Rus for getting some of the top experts to participate and gathering a series of solidly argued clear articles that should allow readers to learn calmly without reserve and without passion about the prospects for the development of artificial intelligence in health.

Let us hope that this book will convince its readers that "there is no question of replacing the doctor with the machine and that the challenge is to organize the natural and collaborative interactions between human expertise and the contributions of artificial intelligence in the daily practice of medicine."[1]

Paris, France                                                        Daniel Couturier
                                              Past Permanent Executive Officer
                                          of the National Academy of Medicine

                                                      Catherine Bréchignac
                                              Past Permanent Executive Officer
                                                  of the Academy of Sciences

---

[1]Villani C., *Donner un sens à l'intelligence artificielle*, p. 197.

# Introduction

Artificial intelligence (AI) is a revolution for some people, fashion for others, and a reality for many aspects of our lives. All areas scientific and otherwise are preparing to experience the upheavals it will inevitably bring.

At the forefront of scientific fields awaiting this impact is health. On the one hand, there are the usual problems such as diagnostic errors, variability of situations, fallibility of experts, and great difficulties in transmitting research information to practitioners. On the other hand, AI excels at digesting piles of literature, finding rare correlations, and analyzing images and other data that are ever more numerous produced by medicine, a field in which the stakes are of course literally vital.

This book provides an overview of AI in medicine and, more generally, looks at issues at the intersection of mathematics, informatics, and medicine. It reaches out to AI experts by offering hindsight and a global vision, and to non-experts intrigued by this timely and important subject. It provides clear, objective, and reasonable information on issues at this intersection avoiding any fantasies that the AI topic may evoke. The book provides a broad kaleidoscopic viewpoint rather than deep technical details.

The book was gradually compiled by the Artificial Intelligence and Health working group created by the National Academy of Medicine and the Academy of Sciences of France at our suggestion. The sessions of the working group were an opportunity for us to explore the questions we had asked ourselves during our meeting at the Ethics Council of the Epidemium competition. Above all, they were a means of inviting recognized specialists to contribute and collaborate such as mathematicians, modelers and analysts, data scientists, statisticians, oncologists, surgeons, oncogeneticists, sociologists, hospital administrators, and lawyers.

For the applications of AI to be impactful a multidisciplinary approach is required. This is the reason we set up a multidisciplinary working group with specialists from various fields of medicine, mathematics, and computation. Our conversations were fruitful because we were able to discuss topics that are intrinsically multidisciplinary with experts representing all their medical and computational aspects. The dialogue of this think tank made us realize that the doctors of the future will have to be "multilingual" in medicine, data, and computation. This will require new approaches to training medical students, something we believe should be done early in medical training.

The road ahead is full of challenges, but the journey is worth it. The "mechanical" medical doctor (MD) is certainly not for tomorrow and certainly not desirable. The doctor of the future should be "augmented," better equipped, and well informed to prevent, analyze, decide, and treat disease with empathy and the human touch. The aim will be to improve diagnoses, observations, therapeutic choices, and outcomes.

Imaging and, more generally, the analysis of medical data will benefit from AI and machine learning advances. Medicine is an area of choice for the full exploitation of images because medical image details are too fine or subtle to be picked up by the naked eye. Additionally, when image resolution is poor, algorithms can identify the missing data and enhance image quality. Mathematical models can then be used to predict future outcomes given the current images.

Modeling can be used as an enhanced tool for the evaluation of chemotherapy treatments. Right now tumor response to chemotherapy is estimated using approximate measurements of the diameter of the tumor. New advances in tumor growth modeling processes make it possible to predict tumor response to treatments that take into account macroscopic features. Equally important is the consideration of tumor genomic data or modeling. In the future these predictions will take into account information at both the molecular and the macroscopic scale and will be a significant challenge.

The correspondence between genotype and phenotype remains the most vexing of the mysteries of biology, but new statistical learning methods offer a workaround. They enable the analysis of extraordinary molecular datasets to be self-mathematized to better identify the regions of the genome associated with tumor progression and determine the most appropriate treatment. This same machine learning approach can help to overcome the imbalance between the large number of variables studied and the small sample sizes available by selecting the most relevant data. The future of clinical research will be enabled by tumor databanks. Combining clinical and biological data stored in tumor banks will likely become standard practice for clinical research. Clinical trials are in the process of being renewed: the platforms that make it possible to record and cross-reference large clinical and molecular data suggest new trial formats. Studies target molecular abnormalities more than organs. When strong pilot alterations are identified, molecular information will gradually enter into common practice.

Pathology will also be renewed by AI. Today pathologists depend on physical slides that cannot be shared. Imaging the slides will in future lead to pathology databanks. Such virtual slides will allow remote analysis without a microscope. Multiparametric analysis makes it possible to search for increasingly complex information. New technologies for organ exploration that are extremely promising are beginning to emerge yielding large amounts of data, in addition. The microbiota, the environment, and now entire ecosystems can be identified by statistical tools.

Finally, and perhaps most importantly, medical data are becoming accessible, especially to young multidisciplinary teams working in open mode (open science, open data).

Such developments will have to face up to major challenges associated with the race for the three major ingredients that are the object of unbridled competition worldwide: human expert brains, high-performance computer equipment, and very large multiparameter datasets.

First of all is the challenge of finding human expert brains. AI is mainly carried out by experts endowed with a spirit of collaboration, ready to take on a challenge, and with expertise in interdisciplinary contacts. Dual-competency profiles for new jobs (health and Big Data, algorithms and medicine, etc.) are very popular, yet the talent pool is scant. Training a new generation of scientists ready to occupy these interfaces is a major challenge. There are not enough trainers or programs; we will have to start new experimental training programs.

Next is the challenge of producing high-performance computer equipment. Europe lags behind the United States and China in terms of investment. The AI of health in the future will require large storage and computing centers, some of which will be internal and some will be outsourced.

Last but not least is the search for machine learning algorithms to identify correlations, regularities, and weak signals. This will require very large multiparameter datasets, labeled data, and cross-referencing the data of various sources (private and public) whose marriage can only be accomplished with governmental support. In France the largest existing public health databases are interlinked such as SNIIRAM (National Information System Inter Plans Health Insurance), SNDS (National Health Data System), and hospital platforms such as the platform of the AP-HP (Administration of Paris Public Hospitals). They are all intended to be part of a larger entity aimed at facilitating their access for research purposes.

The construction of such large medical datasets presents a triple challenge. First, the technical and technological challenge posed by the size of the data has to be resolved. This includes rapid access to data, handling a variety of formats, addressing the considerable number of imperfections in the data, and the need for enhanced cybersecurity. Second, the ethical and legal challenge relating to the protection of personal data requires solutions that ensure public confidence. Third, trust in sharing data is difficult to come by in practice since it requires convincing data owners to overcome their reluctance to join forces. In the French context the State is playing a key role in all these areas. France has set up the Health Data Hub to facilitate research.

Finally, patients will have to play their part in such developments. This includes giving informed consent, participating in the development of tools, and contributing to the evolution of practices and mentalities. While physicians retain responsibility for contact with and explanations to patients, an interaction between humans and algorithms in medicine that is appropriate and constructive is likely to emerge (especially defined for the human dimension).

Today, all nations aspiring to be part of the global innovation scene are embarking on AI and health programs. The United States and China have announced national strategies to stimulate the development and applications of AI with medicine and healthcare as important pillars. France is no exception as shown by releasing the report "Giving meaning to artificial intelligence" (by Cédric Villani) in March 2018. The findings in the report are the result of six months of interdisciplinary work including many hearings. This report outlines a strategy for a coordinated AI policy in France and, more broadly, in Europe. The President of the French Republic adopted most of the recommendations in his speech on March 29, 2018.

The multidisciplinary working group responsible for the genesis of this book contributed some of the background and reflections that shaped the report sent to the government; it also influenced details of the Data Protection Act that adapts French law for the purposes of the EU General Data Protection Regulation (RGPD). It is intended to provoke advance thinking of both specialists and the merely curious. This book brings together a variety of very brief contributions proposed by stakeholders to the working group. All the themes already outlined are included.

The last part of this book examines breakthroughs that connect medicine and society such as the ambivalent role of new modes of information (particularly, social networks that disrupt communication and spread fake news and conspiracy theories), the emotional and sometimes misleading dialogue between humans and machines, and humanity's temptation to push ahead without safeguards. Throughout the book, contributors emphasize directions and dominant themes more than details.

The purpose of this book is to give the reader an overview of the state of the art of AI in medicine by providing examples and suggestions of how the medical field will change. Machines supporting and augmenting doctors should not be seen as scary. Rather, the future "augmented" doctor will provide patients with better and more personalized treatments.

Bernard Nordlinger  
Cédric Villani  
Daniela Rus

# Contents

## Diagnosis and Treatment Assistance

## Research

# Editors and Contributors

## About the Editors

**Bernard Nordlinger** Professor of Surgical Oncology, Université de Versailles, AP-HP; Coorganizer of the IA and Health Working Group of the Académie nationale de Médecine and Académie des sciences.

**Cédric Villani** mathematician; Fields Medal winner; professor at the Claude Bernard Lyon 1 University; member of the Academy of Sciences; Member of the French Parliament; first Vice President of the Office parlementaire d'évaluation des choix scientifiques et technologiques (OPECST).

**Daniela Rus** Director of the Computer Science and Artificial Intelligence Laboratory (CSAIL); Andrew and Erna Viterbi Professor in the Department of Electrical Engineering and Computer Science (EECS) at the Massachusetts Institute of Technology.

## Contributors

**Nicholas Ayache** Research Director, INRIA, Sophia Antipolis, Member of the Academy of Sciences. Scientific Director of the AI institute "3IA Côte d'Azur".

**Emmanuel Bacry** Senior Researcher at CNRS, University of Paris-Dauphine, Chief Scientific Director Health Data Hub, Head of Health/Data projects, École Polytechnique.

**Cécile Badoual** Department of Pathology, University of Paris Descartes, Georges Pompidou European Hospital, APHP.

**Ran D. Balicer, M.D., Ph.D., MPH** Director, Clalit Research Institute, Director, Health Policy Planning Department, Clalit Health Services, Chief Physician office, Associate Professor, Epidemiology Depart- ment, Faculty of Health Sciences, Ben-Gurion University of the Negev.

**Martine Ben Amar** Professor of Physics, Laboratory of Physics, École normale supérieure et Sorbonne University; Institute of Cancerology of Sorbonne University.

**Mehdi Benchoufi** Faculty of Medicine, University of Paris Descartes, INSERM UMR1153, Centre d'Épidémiologie Clinique, Hôpital Hôtel Dieu, AP-HP, coordinator of the Epidemium program.

**Jean-Yves Blay** Director General of the Léon Bérard Centre, Groupe Sarcome Français, NETSARC+, EURACAN, Centre de Recherche en Cancérologie de Lyon, LYRI- CAN, Université Claude Bernard, Lyon 1.

**Jeanne Bossi-Malafosse** Lawyer specializing in personal data and health information systems, DELSOL Lawyers.

**Pierre Bougnères** Pediatric Endocrinologist, Professor of Pediatrics at the University of Paris-Sud, Inserm Unit U1169 "Gene Therapy, Genetics, Epigenetics in Neurology, Endocrinology and Child Development".

**Charles Bouveyron** Professor of Applied Mathematics, Inria Chair in Data Science, Laboratoire J.A. Dieudonné, UMR CNRS 735, Equipe Epione, INRIA Sophia Antipolis, Université Côte d'Azur, Nice, France.

**Johan Brag** Chief Scientific Officer, Median Technologies, Valbonne, France.

**Gérald Bronner** Professor of Sociology, University of Paris 7, Académie des Technologies, Académie nationale de Médecine.

**Jurgi Camblong** CEO and Co-founder of SOPHiA GENETICS, member of the Council for Digital Transformation, Swiss Federal Government.

**Chandra Cohen-Stavi** Clalit Research Institute.

**Thierry Colin** Senior Vice-President, Radiomics Business Area, SOPHiA GENETICS.

**Christel Daniel, M.D., Ph.D.** Deputy Director of the Data and Digital Innovations Departement—Information Systems DirectionAP-HP, LIMICS INSERM UMRS 1142.

**Laurent Degos** Academy of Medicine. Academy of Sciences (correspondent) Professor Emeritus University of Paris. Former President of the High Authority of Health.

**Laurence Devillers** Professor of Artificial Intelligence and Ethics, Sorbonne-Université/LIMSI-CNRS, member of CERNA-Allistène, DATAIA mission member, founding member of HUB France IA, IEEE P7008 Nudging member.

**Olivier de Fresnoye** Coordinator of the Epidemium programme. Ozanan Meireles, surgeon, MGH.

**Mostafa El Hajjam** Interventional Radiologist, Department of IMAGERIE, Ambroise Paré Hospital, Boulogne.

**Stephane Gaïffas** LPMA Professor, University of Paris-Diderot. Christine Garcia, IBM France, consultant and teacher, member of Syntec Numérique Santé.

**Christine Garcia** IBM France, consultant and teacher, member of Syntec Numérique Santé.

**Claude Gissot** CNAM, Director of Strategy, Studies and Statistics.

**Marcel Goldberg** Epidemiologist, Emeritus Professor at University of Paris Descartes.

**Matthieu Grall** Head of the technological expertise department of the Commission Nationale de l'Informatique et des Libertés.

**Jean-Patrick Lajonchère** Managing Director of the Paris Saint-Joseph Hospital Group, chargé de mission to the Minister of Europe and Foreign Affairs for export health support.

**Catherine Cheze Le Rest, M.D.,** Professor in Biophysics, Department of Nuclear Medicine, University of Poitiers.

**Alain Livartowski** Oncologist, Institut Curie—Ensemble hospitalier, Deputy Director of the Data Department, member of the Institut du Thorax.

**Bertrand Lukacs** Urologist, Paris.

**Ozanan R. Meireles** Surgeon, MGH

**Nicolas Padoy** Associate Professor on a Chair of Excellence and head of research group CAMMA (Computational Analysis and Modeling of Medical Activities) in the ICube laboratory at University of Strasbourg.

**Jean-Yves Robin** Chairman of LMB Venture, Vice President of the National Federation of Third Party Trusted Numbers, former Director of ASIP Santé.

**Bertrand Rondepierre** Armament engineer, now at Google.

**Jacques Rouessé** Medical oncologist, honorary director of the Centre René-Huguenin de lutte contre le cancer, member of the Aca- démie nationale de Médecine.

**Daniela Rus** Director of the Computer Science and Artificial Intelligence Laboratory (CSAIL), and Andrew and Erna Viterbi Professor in the Department of Electrical Engineering and Computer Science (EECS) at the Massachusetts Institute of Technology.

**Elisa Salamanca** Director of the Data and Digital Innovations Departement—Information Systems Direction, AP-HP.

**François Sigaux** Professor of Haematoloy, University of Paris Diderot—APHP; Executive Scientific Director of CEA's Fundamental Research.

**Georges Uzbelger** IBM France, mathematician and teacher, member of the Syntec Numérique Santé.

**Guy Vallancien** Member of the National Academy of Medicine, Member of the Parliamentary Office for Scientific and Technological Choices, President of CHAM.

**Alain-Jacques Valleron** Epidemiologist, Professor Emeritus of Biostatistics and Medical Informatics at Sorbonne University, Member of the Academy of Sciences, Inserm Unit U1169 "Genetic Therapy, Genetics, Epigenetics in Neurology, Endocrinology and Child Development".

**Jean-Philippe Vert** Mathematician, Specialist in artificial intelligence and bioinformatics, research scientist at Google and adjunct professor at MINES ParisTech and École normale supérieure.

**Cédric Villani** Mathematician, Fields Medal winner, professor at the Claude Bernard Lyon 1 University, member of the Academy of Sciences, Member of French Parliament, first Vice-President of the Office parlementaire d'évaluation des choix scientifiques et technologiques (OPECST).

**Dimitris Visvikis** Physicist, Director of Research INSERM, LaTIM, UMR 1101, Fellow IPEM, Senior Member IEEE.

**Gilles Wainrib** Scientific Director and co-founder of Owkin.

**Marie Zins** Epidemiologist, University of Paris Descartes, Director of the Population Epidemiological Cohorts Unit (UMS 011 Inserm-UVSQ), in charge of the Constances National Infrastructure Biology and Health.

# Artificial Intelligence and Tomorrow's Health

**Cédric Villani and Bertrand Rondepierre**

The potential of artificial intelligence (AI) in the field of health is immense and has been, from the very beginning of the discipline, subject to significant work since the beginning of the 20th century. The 1970s saw an explosion in the scientific community's interest in biomedical applications helped by the availability of distributed computing resources such as SUMEX-AIM (Stanford University Medical Experimental Computer for Artificial Intelligence in Medicine) from Stanford University and Rutgers University. Among the first practical applications to be identified was the MYCIN project. Developed in the 1960s and 1970s at Stanford University it used an expert system to identify bacteria that cause serious infections and then provided appropriate treatments.

In addition to the obvious benefits for society as a whole, the field of health has always exercised a particular fascination in the scientific community in addition to being a natural playground for artificial intelligence. The general increase in the volumes of data available in extraordinary proportions and the complexity, number, and variety of phenomena involved make health an almost infinite and extremely diversified subject of study. This complexity, which a priori defeats any attempt to fully model human biology and the mechanisms at work, is precisely the privileged place of expression for AI. Like a doctor, AI techniques are based on observations that produce information that can be used by the practitioner when confronted with theoretical and empirical knowledge. In a context where it is increasingly difficult to replicate the results of community-driven studies and where, as in many other areas, the transition from discovery to a product or new practice is rarely frictionless, AI is an exception because it is perceived as a capacity that can be directly activated and used in the field.

C. Villani
Assemblée Nationale, Paris, France
e-mail: cedric.Villani@assemblee-nationale.fr

B. Rondepierre (✉)
now at Google, Paris, France

© Springer Nature Switzerland AG 2020
B. Nordlinger et al. (eds.), *Healthcare and Artificial Intelligence*,
https://doi.org/10.1007/978-3-030-32161-1_1

However, the need for theoretical knowledge is sometimes challenged by recent approaches, such as neural networks and deep learning, that manage to discover for themselves how to accomplish certain tasks without a priori information on the phenomenon under study. Based on the observation of many examples, these methods establish correlational links between the patterns observed and the ability to perform the task requested. However, such discovered links can be misleading because of the well-known difference between correlation and causality that mathematicians know well, on the one hand, and because data can carry biases that distort the relevance of the result obtained, on the other hand. Such weaknesses are not critical when it comes to recommending a movie but can have particularly disastrous consequences in the field of medicine. Autonomous discovery by algorithms is not a necessity, however, because centuries of study and deepening our knowledge of medicine have enabled us to produce a wide spectrum of models applicable to human biology unlike in some fields where human beings are perfectly incapable of explaining the cognitive processes at work to translate data into usable information. If these models exist, it must be noted that medicine as a whole remains to be based on observation and its practice is therefore extremely dependent on the experience of the practitioner whose diagnosis is based on a priori knowledge, as well as on a history of previous situations with which the new one is compared. Two practitioners in health and AI with different experiences will therefore potentially and naturally arrive at two different diagnoses from the same observation.

Like some therapeutic or epidemiological discoveries whose explanation escapes the current state of our knowledge some phenomena are only understood through an empirical process. Thus, it is at the intersection between the blind approach and full formal modeling that AI can reveal its true potential and, for example, avoid gross errors that are incomprehensible to a human being.

The importance of empirical information leads to the observation that the data that express it, even more than elsewhere, constitute the core of the practice of medicine in its relationship with the patient. It is therefore not surprising that there is an exponential increase in the quantity and diversity of available data as part of a global digitization of all medical practice and the use of ever more numerous and varied sensors. Reports written by health professionals, analytical results, genomics, medical imaging, biological signal recordings, and drug use history are examples of data sources that can be the raw material for AI research. Their diversity is an expression of the multiplicity of possible applications for health some of which can be cited as recurrent examples: diagnostic assistance, pharmacovigilance, materiovigilance, infectiovigilance, personalized medicine, patient follow-up, clinical research, and medical–administrative uses. However, the data are not in themselves an "open sesame" whose possession alone will allow the development of AI. Data in themselves are only of interest if they are clean, neat, and well labeled. It is for this reason that any AI approach necessarily involves a work step on these data to extract the essence of the data and thus enable them to be exploited at their true value.

The state of the art of AI for these various applications is highly heterogeneous. Like other fields, neural networks have made significant progress in the exploitation of biological signals as evidenced by the success of young French companies such as

Cardiologs, which specializes in the automatic analysis of electrocardiograms. On these issues the combination of data availability and algorithm refinement has made it possible to match, if not sometimes exceed, the level of performance obtained by a human to detect pathologies from these signals. Similarly, use of such signals related to vigilance have been made possible with initial successes (particularly, in the correlation of pathologies) thanks to the depth of public databases. One example is the work published in February 2018 in *The Lancet Public Health* showing that excessive alcohol consumption is associated with a tripling of the risk for dementia, in general, and a doubling of the risk for developing Alzheimer disease. Advances in natural language processing have made it possible to make progress in the extraction of information (particularly, from reports written by doctors) and one hopefully to capitalize on medical information in the long term by simplifying the upstream work of qualifying and enriching data. The AI revolution for health has only just begun, and the coming years should be rich in new developments.

Key to the success of this revolution is the confluence of three types of resources: human, empirical (through databases), and computational (since it is primarily about large-scale computing). The human resource is the most critical of this triptych and the most protean. It is primarily critical to expertise in the field of AI and in the field of health and exerts real tension on profiles displaying this double competence. Experts with such competence are particularly valued not only for their ability to inject medical knowledge into AI methods, but also for the reciprocal aim of bringing AI closer to the medical professions by matching them to the most relevant needs and uses. Human resources are also critical to getting professionals and patients fully involved. Since data and their qualification are a major concern, as well as materializing the link between machines and the real world, they cannot do without those who produce data, those who enrich data to associate data with a business value, or those who exploit data in their medical practice.

The battle for AI is being fought on many levels. This is especially true of the health sector where many countries are trying to address the issue and position themselves as leaders. First, a battle for human resources is being fought in parallel between countries, between companies and the State, and between companies. Second, there is a struggle for leadership in AI for health. At first glance, the United States appears to be in front with a definite lead, while Canada, the United Kingdom, and Israel are positioning themselves as very serious competitors. Israel's case is particularly interesting in this regard. Gathering its own data through a systematic and authoritative campaign involving doctors and the entire hospital community means the initial resource necessary for a larger scale AI approach to health has already been constituted. Moreover, research teams have been developed within a few large insurance funds that are leading the entire social security apparatus and capable of setting up ingenious models based largely on interdisciplinarity and cooperation between specialties.

## French Strengths and Weaknesses

For its part France is already in a privileged position to play an important role internationally in the field of AI for health. French higher education and research have always occupied a prominent place at the international level, particularly because of the recognized excellence of scientific training in France. Excellence, particularly in mathematics and computer science, gives France a competitive advantage as confirmed by the presence of many French people at the head of many prestigious companies and teams working on AI. Yann LeCun is the most famous of them and a leading figure on neural networks. He is currently working at both New York University and Facebook AI Research (FAIR). Expanding the definition of the French community to include the Francophone community we must also mention Yoshua Bengio, another leading figure in the field playing a major part in the Canadian strategy. While this academic excellence is the sine qua non condition necessary to occupy an advantageous position in a tough international competition, it is not sufficient to guarantee it. Globally, the current rigidity of medical training remains a problem today since it will not be able to meet the need for multidisciplinarity that will only increase. The integration of AI and, more broadly, digital technology into curricula is a must for professions that will be at the forefront of such technological developments.

Downstream of research and contrary to certain preconceived ideas innovation in France remains very dynamic despite little publicity and visibility. While a significant proportion of the scientific publications of digital giants are relayed both in the specialized press and in national and even international dailies, some French successes, such as Therapixel (winner of a world competition against teams from the world's largest laboratories), remain unpublicized. Even if France is not the base of any digital giant, it is not deprived from an industrial point of view since it is home to heavyweights in the field such as Sanofi or Atos (which have a more transverse position) and OVH (which provides advanced cloud-computing services).

Academic, entrepreneurial, and industrial forces are therefore well represented and can rely on data resources that are unique in the healthcare field all over the world. Indeed, France's Jacobin tradition has led it over time to set up a health system that collects, but not exclusively, the data necessary for the performance of medical and administrative tasks in a mode that is essentially centralized and managed by the State. Moreover, more than 65 million French people participate in this system giving it the critical size necessary. So, it is conceivable that the use of already capitalized data will lead to short-term successes. These data are grouped together in the National Health Data System (NSDS), which now has as its primary objective the organization and implementation of healthcare reimbursement.

The sensitivity of the domain and the information that is manipulated raises the question of trust in a more singular way. In this context the fact that the public health task is essentially carried out by the State or by structures that report directly to it makes developing AI in health and structuring organizations for this purpose a legitimate intermediary of trust. The challenge here is to ensure that the need for such developments is accepted and to guarantee the framework within which they will be carried out without the use of intermediaries, although the latter are not exempt from obligations either. Indeed, the existence of French and European regulations (the EU General Data Protection Regulation or RGPD) as a spearhead contributes to creating a framework of trust favorable to the development of AI systems that respect and protect individuals and are therefore all the more likely to be successful and accepted by French citizens.

These comparative advantages will not be the only determinants of French success. Competition for human resources could lead to French research laboratories and companies drying up and becoming a breeding ground for non-European players. As a result, the dynamics of innovation would be jeopardized permanently undermining French ability to excel in this area. Moreover, because of the difficulty of conducting research projects in the health sector due to administrative and regulatory complexities there remains an entry barrier that does not allow major players, whether academic or industrial, to emerge.

While the NSDS is considered an immense asset, it is nonetheless limited and insufficient to allow the development of a real French force for AI and health on its own. A system that has been designed solely for medical and administrative purposes cannot be expected to be naturally equipped to support and promote an efficient research and innovation approach in the field of AI. To this end there is a very pragmatic lack not only of the necessary hardware and software resources to implement such an approach, but also of the governance and organization necessary to ensure coherence at the national level. This is evidenced by customer data available in hospitals to date still not being shared with national data. Even under the first NSDS implementation it may take months or even years for data to be capitalized within the system when it has not yet been coded for reimbursement. As data quality is essential it must be borne in mind that a great deal of work will be needed to make data directly usable by AI approaches and that data management will have to be accompanied by governance that is currently structurally lacking.

Finally, excellence in AI, health research, and innovation on their own is not enough to create economic champions. Whatever the quality of upstream work it must be associated with the existence of a large market that does not yet exist either within the State, with private companies, or with French citizens. If we agree that the market is at a minimum European and even possibly international, then there is still a chasm to be crossed to transform innovation into economic success (especially with French venture capital remaining insufficient to face international competition).

## A Project for France

Whatever the plan to be implemented it is important to keep in mind the three main types of challenges that any approach will face: technical; legal and ethical; and trust and organization. Technical challenges essentially constitute the ability to deploy new technologies in adapted systems while ensuring the continuity and recovery of existing systems. These challenges exist whatever the underlying technology and are the result of meticulous architectural work. However, the legal and ethical challenges raised are much more specific to AI and to the field of application of health because the criticality and sensitivity of the application require a particular investigation. Finally, the challenges of trust and organization reveal that the first obstacle to the development of AI is not so much technological or regulatory as it is human. AI cannot develop without the trust of its users and the support of organizations that are often ill-equipped to deal with such a broad and cross-cutting issue. Contrary to popular belief it would seem that technical challenges are often easier to meet than anticipated, while trust and organizational challenges are much more difficult to address than expected. This is certainly explained by the fact that a technical challenge usually requires a technical solution, while a human challenge requires much more in-depth work, reflection, and pedagogy.

To organize French action in this area the report "For a meaningful artificial intelligence" proposes a global approach aimed at establishing a system of both academic and industrial scope in the field of AI and health by capitalizing on French strengths. The first requirement for such an approach is to set a direction with some ambitious objectives of general interest to maintain and structure the system effort over time. Clearly identifying these objectives is also a prerequisite to equipping them since such action will certainly not be the same if we are interested in reducing the risk of nosocomial disease or in personalized medicine. Setting a direction is also an opportunity to lead upstream reflections on ethics and trust by integrating them into concrete projects thus avoiding the pitfall of overly theoretical discussions that could lead to decisions to the detriment of progress, even though the apparently contradictory dimensions of these projects were reconcilable.

Before others do it for the country it is essential to reorganize the French health system along the lines of the one that led to the success of the digital economy (i.e., the platform model as an intermediary in accessing information, content, services, and goods published or provided by third parties). Such a platform is an opportunity to deploy state-of-the-art computing and data storage resources compatible with the uses of AI. This technical aspect is more a prerequisite and an update of the existing system than a breakthrough in itself. However, it is the vector that will have to collect the data relevant to the uses of AI in health, to instrument their collection, and to capture data in real time. In doing so this platform is intended to be deployed from the central level to the local level (hospitals, health professionals, and patients) thus bringing together systems that have historically been disconnected from each other. From an economic point of view it is a means of changing the situation by allowing third parties (researchers, contractors, large companies, and public authorities) to develop and experiment with new functionalities that are directly based on the health system and the data it contains. Thus, the platform opens up a new way of creating and distributing added value.

Emphasis should be placed on research and experimentation. Complaints are recurrent as a result of too heavy regulatory obligations and too long delays in the investigation of cases. While the situation has improved considerably in recent years, to be compatible with the pace of innovation the introduction of "sandboxes" in the health sector that are open to experimentation would temporarily ease the constraints on stakeholders, support them in fulfilling their obligations, and carry out experiments under real conditions. Research will also be the first beneficiary of this policy. Thanks to privileged access to data and flexible experimental conditions, such public research laboratories as the interdisciplinary institutes for research in artificial intelligence (3IA institutes) proposed to free the forces of our academic fabric, should find fertile ground here for the development of AI for tomorrow's health.

Finally, the most significant difficulty will be posed by organizational challenges that will involve setting up a governance system with a cross functional data policy whose objective would be to think upstream in terms of data collection, data capitalization, and governance of the health platform, as well as organization of the effort around the development of AI. A project such as the Shared Medical Record should be accompanied by an AI dimension to be explored in the project so that data are no longer capitalized only for documentary purposes, but also for subsequent research, innovation, and exploitation within the scope of AI. Such a possibility requires specific structuring so that the patient's history can be followed, an operation made difficult today since the use of NIR[1] is not systematic. Of the conditions necessary for success it should be stressed that development of the AI skills of organizations (companies, administrations, regulatory authorities, doctors, and health professionals) is essential. The same is true of patients where the need to demystify AI is becoming increasingly important to avoid a feeling of mistrust or refusal to take advantage of the opportunities offered by these technologies. Acculturation, acceptance, and trust must each be a primary concern since the development of AI depends mainly on patient involvement.

## European Tracks

It is generally accepted that France has not reached the level in terms of AI needed to compete against such giants as the United States or China and must look instead to Europe. In the health field, working directly at the EU scale is a hard task to undertake. Although it would have been natural to cooperate with Germany, it has a much more heterogeneous and disparate health system than that of France and therefore does not offer the same opportunities in the short term. There seem to be so many different situations in the various Member States that now would be a good time to carry out a survey, map the different European health systems, and establish the potentialities in terms of AI. Depending on the results of such a study the desirability or otherwise of developing a European health system deploying the logic of the French plan on a European scale could be evaluated. That could support the French academic and industrial policy of AI applied to health.

---

[1] Registration number or social security number in France.

It will only be as a result of major changes that France will be able through the European Union to seize the position it wishes to occupy in the world in terms of AI and health.

# Advancing Healthcare Through Data-Driven Medicine and Artificial Intelligence

Ran D. Balicer and Chandra Cohen-Stavi

*If it were not for the great variability among individuals,
medicine might as well be a science, not an art.*
Sir William Osler, 1892.

## Introduction: The Status Quo and Its Toll

Health systems have been facing escalating challenges in recent decades since the increase in demand and costs cannot be met by a similar rate of increase in human resource and invested capital. The rise in demand is the result of several key trends: the population is growing older, and the relative proportion of the population over the age of 65 is rapidly increasing. As the average healthcare needs of the elderly population are far greater than those of the younger population this trend is straining healthcare systems. In parallel, chronic disease morbidity in all age groups is becoming increasingly more prevalent. A majority of people above the age of 50 years have chronic disease comorbidity or multimorbidity (i.e., two diseases or more), and this multimorbidity has a synergistic impact on their healthcare needs.

Such strained systems and individual providers are working in an ineffective and error-prone traditional model of reactive care. In the current state of affairs the intuitive and experience-based art of medicine is failing us and allows for substandard care to be the norm, even in the most advanced healthcare systems. It has been estimated that 45% of the evidence-based interventions required in routine care are missed, and

R. D. Balicer (✉) · C. Cohen-Stavi
Clalit Research Institute, Clalit Health Services, Tel Aviv, Israel
e-mail: rbalicer@gmail.com

R. D. Balicer
Faculty of Health Sciences, Public Health Department, Ben-Gurion University of the Negev, Beersheba, Israel

© Springer Nature Switzerland AG 2020
B. Nordlinger et al. (eds.), *Healthcare and Artificial Intelligence*,
https://doi.org/10.1007/978-3-030-32161-1_2

many deaths are the result of medical errors or inappropriate care,[1] despite clinical professionals doing their best to deliver the right care. Increased complexity in the options of care models, medical treatments, and medical technologies bring about intensifying challenges in disentangling the evidence for effectiveness, with almost 2.5 million English-language articles per year published in scientific journals.[2] The providers themselves bear severe professional and personal cost for this continuous increase in workload and inappropriately designed work setting, with recent surveys suggesting that up to 50% of physicians reporting severe burnout signs and symptoms.[3]

## The Promise of Artificial Intelligence in Transforming Healthcare for the Better

It has been suggested that healthcare systems must adapt and profoundly change in their operating model to allow sustainable effective care to their members in view of these basic inadequacies and escalating challenges. One way to navigate rising healthcare demand and exponentially increasing complexity in care and treatment options is to proactively anticipate future demand, risks, and health needs and use this knowledge for better care allocation and patient-centered treatment decisions. The ability to understand the dynamic factors affecting health through data analytics, pattern detection, and prediction is paramount to creating more intelligent healthcare.

Effective and efficient models of care must strive to be proactive and prevention focused rather than reactive and treatment focused; integrated rather than divided into detached care silos; precise and tailored to the specific patient's unique set of characteristics and needs rather than based on average population observations. It is a common wisdom that the smart use of data in healthcare is both a key requisite and driving force to allow such changes to be implemented on a large scale.

The expansion of embedded information technology (IT) systems across healthcare settings provides an increasing wealth of data that can be harnessed through advanced analytics in a systematic transformation to narrow key gaps for the healthcare systems of the future. These include the widespread implementation of electronic health record systems, the availability of health-related data from personal

---

[1] Makary M.A., Daniel M., "Medical error—the third leading cause of death in the US," 2016. BMJ 2016;353:i2139; Hogan H., Healey F., Neale G. et al., "Preventable deaths due to problems in care in English acute hospitals: A retrospective case record review study," *BMJ Quality and Safety,* 2012.

[2] Ware M., Mabe M., *The STM Report: An Overview of Scientific and Scholarly Journal Publishing,* 2015, The Hague: International Association of Scientific, Technical and Medical Publishers. Retrieved August 7, 2017 from: https://www.stm-assoc.org/2015_02_20_STM_Report_2015.pdf.

[3] Shanafelt T.D., Hasan O., Dyrbye L., Sinsky C., Satele D., Sloan J.O. et al., "Changes in burnout and satisfaction with work-life balance in physicians and the general US working population between 2011 and 2014," *Mayo Clinic Proceedings,* 2015, 90(12), 1600–1613. Medscape survey of 15,000 physicians. Report accessed at: https://www.medscape.com/slideshow/2018-lifestyle-burnout-depression-6009235?faf=1.

and healthcare devices, and the increasing use of genetic testing which produce massive patient-specific datasets. Continuous improvement in computing power and widespread implementation of AI in other daily domains of life increase the drive to implement similar systems in healthcare as well.

Among many opportunities that data and advanced analytics offer for healthcare advancement there is the potential for preventing complications and improving prognosis (to preempt), supporting patient-focused treatment decision-making (to individualize), integrating patient involvement in navigating their care (to align expectations between patients and providers), and the automation of clinical tasks and service allocation to improve the efficiency and safety of health institutions (to make repetitive technical tasks redundant, reduce errors, and reduce clinical variability).

Multiple advanced data analytics techniques are being increasingly used in academic and commercial innovation platforms to develop data-driven tools for the healthcare setting, from basic algorithms based on straightforward regression statistics to the most complex *machine learning* tools based on multiple layers of artificial neural networks. Indeed, most of the computerized solutions in current clinical practice do not rely on independent computer intelligence, but rather on human-generated algorithms based on expertise and research. Still, in this chapter we will loosely use the term artificial intelligence (AI) to denote the wide range of tools that allow computers to perform tasks just as well as if not better than humans.

The National Health Service in the United Kingdom has outlined the ways AI can and is expected to improve and help transform healthcare by allowing for the prediction of individuals who are at risk for illness to target treatment more effectively toward them; the development of AI diagnostic and treatment decision tools tailored to individual need supporting health professionals and patients; and the automation of clinical tasks and service allocation to improve the efficiency and safety of health institutions.[4]

The potential for improvement is profound. It has been shown, for example, that by combining *deep learning* AI techniques with pathologists' diagnoses for identifying metastatic breast cancer an 85% reduction in the human error rate resulted.[5] Such automated analysis has also been shown to find and match specific lung nodules on chest computed tomography scans nearly twice as fast as a panel of radiologists. The power of AI algorithms to diagnose by means of imaging results has been demonstrated in a study in which the performance of algorithms to identify skin cancers was on par with a panel of 21 experts.[6]

---

[4]Harwich E., Laycock K., *Thinking on Its Own: AI in the NHS, 2018*, Reform Research Trust, London, UK.

[5]Wang D., Khosla A., Gargeya R., Irshad H., Beck A.H., "Deep Learning for Identifying Metastatic Breast Cancer," arXiv preprint arXiv:1606.05718, 2016: https://scholar.harvard.edu/humayun/publications/deep-learning-identifying-metastatic-breast-cancer.

[6]Esteva A., Kuprel B., Novoa R.A., Ko J., Swetter S.M., Blau H.M., Thrun S., "Dermatologist-level classification of skin cancer with deep neural network," *Nature*, 2017, 542(7639), 115–118.

AI applications have been ranked based on how likely adoption is and what potential exists for annual savings.[7] AI-assisted robotic surgery was ranked top since it was estimated it could result in fewer complications and errors that would generate a 21% reduction in patient length of stay and $40 billion in annual savings in eight years. The following highest ranked applications were virtual nursing assistants, administrative workflow, fraud detection, and dosage error reduction. Yet very few clinical applications of AI have been realized in practice and research-backed implementations are scarce.

## Artificial Intelligence Implemented in Clinical Practice

In view of the scarcity of clinical AI tool implementation we review two examples of utilizing AI in the clinical setting, both from the Israeli healthcare system, where data and AI have been used in practice for improving clinical care and supporting the transformation discussed above toward more proactive, preventive, precise, and patient-centered care.

Like France, Israel has universal healthcare coverage for all its citizens and provision of care is offered by four health funds. These health funds are public non-profit payer/provider systems that focus on extensive networks of community-based primary and secondary care clinics but that also pay for all inpatient care. As the switching rate between health funds is very low and generally people stay the majority of their life covered under one health fund the organizations have financial interests to maintain their members' health and provide preventive services rather than to increase medical care volume. Israel also benefits from a unique combination of attributes that support healthcare data-driven innovation with two particularly notable attributes. There is an extensive information technology infrastructure of data repositories based on two decades of interoperable electronic health records across inpatient and outpatient settings. These data serve as a platform for data-driven innovation that is rapidly translated into practice. The second is the "start-up nation" culture that exists, which has globally the highest rate of start-ups, venture capital investment, and medical equipment patents per person.[8]

The first example presented reviews an AI implementation toward proactive, predictive prevention. It is well accepted that attempts to address chronic disease in the later phases of overt organ damage and painful dysfunction are limited in their effectiveness and are usually both costly and associated with serious adverse events. If the precursors of pathological processes could accurately be identified at earlier stages, milder interventions would be more effective in delaying or completely averting the deterioration. Patient health data and advanced analytics can be used to predict

---

[7] Kalis B., Collier M., Fu R., "10 promising AI Applications in Health Care," *Harvard Business Review*, May 10, 2018.

[8] Balicer R.D., Afek A., "Digital health nation: Israel's global Big Data innovation hub," *Lancet*, 2017 June 24, 389(10088), 2451–2453.

which patients are expected to undergo acute or chronic slow deterioration toward a preventable outcome or complication allowing proactive preventive intervention.

In aiming to improve clinical prognosis and prevent deterioration to end-stage renal disease (ESRD)—a major costly chronic condition that is a large burden to patients, their families, and the healthcare system—Clalit Health Services, Israel's largest health fund, initiated the planning of a data analytics–driven targeted prevention program in 2010 to reduce the number of ESRD cases through data analytics–driven targeted prevention. It has been shown that patients with early chronic kidney disease can change their expected deterioration path to ESRD through a set of simple preventive interventions. Yet early chronic kidney disease is fairly prevalent and it is usually not feasible in most health systems to reach out to all of these seemingly healthy patients to prevent future illness. Thus, at the Clalit Research Institute a predictive model was developed and continuously impro-ved to identify which Clalit members were at high risk for developing ESRD within a period of five years. Given resource considerations the model targeted 8% of the population in question at highest risk, and that group included nearly 70% of those identified as high risk for future deterioration to ESRD. Clinical action and tailored interventions for this target group of patients were implemented and pri-mary care teams were trained to follow predefined steps once a high-risk patient is among their patient list. Preliminary results of several years of implementation suggest a clinically meaningful drop in the incidence of ESRD among the patients that were targeted for intervention by the model.

This example shows the utility of predictive algorithms to target treatment more effectively toward high-risk patient groups for the prevention of major chronic disease complications. This approach is being applied in other relevant domains to allow for the identification of populations at risk and early identification of impending complications of multiple acute and chronic illnesses.[9]

A second example reviews the development and design of a precise and individualized treatment decision tool. There is great variability among individuals in health-related characteristics, health behaviors, and clinical response to treatment and healthcare systems are ill-equipped to deliver care for such variability.[10] Generally, clinical guidance and action is based on limited evidence of average effects in populations and not based on individualized, patient-specific evidence.[11] This results in patients who need care not getting that care and patients who don't necessarily

[9]Balicer R.D., Cohen C.J., Leibowitz M., Feldman B.S., Brufman I., Roberts C., Hoshen M., "Pneumococcal vaccine targeting strategy for older adults: Customized risk profiling," *Vaccine,* February 12, 2014, 32(8), 990–995; Shadmi E., Flaks-Manov N., Hoshen M., Goldman O., Bitterman H., Balicer R.D., "Predicting 30-day readmissions with preadmission electronic health record data," *Med Care,* March 2015, 53(3), 283–289; Dagan N., Cohen-Stavi C., Leventer-Roberts M., Balicer R.D., "External validation and comparison of three prediction tools for risk of osteoporotic fractures using data from population based electronic health records: Retrospective cohort study," *BMJ,* January 19, 2017, 356, i6755.

[10]Wallace E., Smith S.M., Fahey T., "Variation in medical practice: Getting the balance right," *Family Practice,* 2012.

[11]Yeh R.W., Kramer D.B., "Decision Tools to Improve Personalized Care in Cardiovascular Disease: Moving the Art of Medicine Toward Science," *Circulation,* 2017; 135(12): 1097–1100; Mccartney

need care getting it, or in the selection of the wrong empirical first-line treatment for serious illnesses.

In recent years there has been increasing use of patient-specific data analytics in clinical practice to drive clinical decisions tailored to the person and the affected tissue. These data are mined from medical records and lab tests that generate massive amounts of data (i.e., genetic sequencing). Since many of the frequently discussed examples of precision care focus on use of personal genetic data we will try to focus on using clinical ("phenomic") data to achieve care precision and personalization. We have demonstrated the potential of such data to drive treatment selection recently by analyzing the hypertension treatment SPRINT trial.[12] In this exercise we used data on several thousand participants in a clinical trial called the SPRINT trial. The data were made available to us as part of a global competition (the SPRINT Challenge) run by the *New England Journal of Medicine*.[13]

We have been able to show that while the SPRINT trial summary suggested that high-risk patients with elevated blood pressure should on average have blood pressure treated to a threshold below 120 mmHg, this was not true for a large subgroup of patients in this study. When multiple iterative individual-level modeling (thousands per individual) was performed for each of these trial subjects separately, it was possible to tease out those individuals who would likely suffer the harms of this suggested intensive treatment without experiencing its benefits from those cases that were expected to mainly benefit from this treatment by preventing the complications of uncontrolled blood pressure. This demonstrates the marked impact that individual-level AI-driven decision support may have on every clinical decision faced by physicians in view of their limited capabilities to compile and integrate all the patient's characteristics, the often fragmented and vast amount of clinical data, and the extensive body of clinical evidence that needs to be reconciled.

## Aspirations and Challenges

While the prospects are vast, they are tempered by the limitations and challenges in achieving intelligent health systems including the establishment of adaptable and interoperable infrastructure for sustainable solutions, the issue of the quality and scope of available data, and the multifaceted ethical issues that arise from the use of sensitive data and liabilities related to algorithms used for medical decisions.[14]

---

M., Treadwell J., Maskrey N., Lehman R., "Making Evidence Based Medicine Work for Individual Patients," *BMJ*, 2016, 353:i2452.

[12]Wright J.T. et al. (the SPRINT Research Group), "A Randomized Trial of Intensive Versus Standard Blood-Pressure Control," *N Engl J Med*, December 21, 2017, 377(25), 2506.

[13]Burns N.S., Miller P.W., "Learning What We Didn't Know: The SPRINT Data Analysis Challenge," *N Engl J Med*, June 8, 2017, 376(23), 2205–2207.

[14]Nuffield Council on Bioethics 2018.

Ultimately, the science of data analytics and AI holds much promise, but clinical impact assessment must become more rigorous and the purpose of such scientific efforts must be defined and driven by unmet clinical needs. Uses of AI in practice for clinical decision-making still remain in their infancy and we must wait for early adopters to provide sound evidence on the continuous and sustainable beneficial effects for patient outcomes in a sustained meaningful way. Yet it is our expectation as well as that of many of the current opinion leaders in this field that these applications will realize the promise and make a significant impact to transform healthcare for the better toward more sustainable and effective healthcare systems.

# Artificial Intelligence: A Vector for Positive Change in Medicine

Daniela Rus

Our world has been changing rapidly. Today, telepresence enables students to meet with tutors and doctors to treat patients thousands of miles away. Robots help with packing on factory floors.

Networked sensors enable monitoring of facilities and 3D printing creates customized goods. We are surrounded by a world of possibilities. These possibilities will only get larger as we start to imagine what we can do with advances in artificial intelligence (AI) and robotics.

On the global scale AI will help us generate better insights into addressing some of our biggest challenges: curing diseases by better diagnosing, treating, and monitoring patients; understanding climate change by collecting and analyzing data from vast wireless sensor networks that monitor the oceans, the greenhouse climate, and the condition of plant life; improving governance by data-driven decision-making; eliminating hunger by monitoring, matching, and rerouting supply and demand; and predicting and responding to natural disasters using cyberphysical sensors. It will help us democratize education through massive open online course (MOOC) offerings that are adaptive to student progress and ensure that every child gets access to the skills needed to get a good job and build a great life. It may even help those kids turn their childhood dreams into reality as Iron Man stops being a comic book character and becomes a technological possibility.

At the individual level AI will offer opportunities to make our lives healthier, safer, more convenient, and more satisfying. That means automated cars that can drive us to and from work or prevent life-threatening accidents when our teenagers are at the wheel. It means customized healthcare built using knowledge gleaned from enormous amounts of data. And counter to common knowledge it means more satisfying jobs, not less, as the productivity gains from AI and robotics free us up

D. Rus (✉)
Computer Science and Artificial Intelligence Laboratory (CSAIL), Department of Electrical Engineering and Computer Science (EECS), Massachusetts Institute of Technology, Cambridge, USA
e-mail: rus@csail.mit.edu

© Springer Nature Switzerland AG 2020
B. Nordlinger et al. (eds.), *Healthcare and Artificial Intelligence*,
https://doi.org/10.1007/978-3-030-32161-1_3

from monotonous tasks and let us focus on the creative, social, and high-end tasks that computers are incapable of.

All these things—and so much more—become possible when we direct the power of computing to solve the world's most challenging problems. Advances are happening in three different but overlapping fields: robotics, *machine learning*, and artificial intelligence. Robotics puts computing into motion and gives machines autonomy. AI adds intelligence giving machines the ability to reason. *Machine learning* cuts across both robotics and AI and enables machines to learn, improve, and make predictions. Progress is being made quickly in each of these fields, so let me pause for a moment and tell you what's already happening today.

Robots have already become our partners in both industrial and domestic settings. They work side-by-side with people in assembly plants building cars and many other goods. They help surgeons perform difficult procedures improving outcomes and reducing scars. They mow our lawns, vacuum our floors, and even milk our cows. Researchers are making strides in improving what robots can do. Most car manufacturers have announced self-driving car projects that will employ sensors to give vehicles a much better sense of road conditions than we can get with the naked eye. This technology will significantly reduce road fatalities through safe driving in the upcomming years.

Other industry sectors will also benefit from this technology. For example, my team at MIT's Computer Science and Artificial Intelligence Lab (CSAIL) is testing an ingestible robot that will enable incision-free surgery.[1] The patient swallows a robot packaged within an ice pill. When the pill reaches the stomach, the ice dissolves, the robot deploys, and can then be controlled by surgeons using programmable magnetic fields to do tasks such as removing foreign objects, collecting tissue samples, patching internal wounds, or delivering medicine to precise locations. As ingestible robots improve, I believe we'll be able to offer new surgical alternatives that are less invasive, less painful, and have much lower risk of infection. Looking farther down the road this technology could intersect with advances in genetics and sequencing and even lead to the ability to swallow a pill containing the right cells and biological agents to self-heal or grow a new internal organ. Medical advances are only one potential area of application. We're also building robots with the strength and agility to replace humans in emergency situations and dangerous terrains, possibly even in space.

In addition to the physical capabilities being demonstrated by robots rapid advances are being made in enabling how much information machines can process. *Machine learning* refers to a process that starts with a body of data and then tries to derive a rule or procedure that explains the data or predicts future data. *Machine learning* algorithms have potential applications in any field that has to process a lot of data. Medicine is a great example. Researchers have developed a predictive model that looks at thousands of data points and models different subtypes of lymphoma to diagnose cancer. This new AI-based approach was tasked with reviewing images of lymph node cells to diagnose cancer. On its own the system had an error rate of

---

[1]http://news.mit.edu/2016/ingestible-origami-robot-0512.

7.5%, worse than the 3.5% rate of human pathologists.[2] However, when both the AI system and the pathologist reviewed the data the error rate went down to only 0.5%. Today such systems may be deployed in the world's most advanced cancer treatment centers. But, imagine a future where every practitioner—even those working in small practices in rural settings—had access to this technology. An overworked doctor may not have the time to review every new study and clinical trial, but working in tandem with AI systems the doctors will offer their patients the most cutting-edge diagnosis and treatment options.

Researchers have also developed a digital pen that measures movement 80 times a second to detect and diagnose dementia and Parkinson disease more accurately than we can today. They're even investigating a method of manipulating metabolic pathways that may hold the secret to reversing human obesity.

*Machine learning* is powering many other services: product recommendations, prevention of money laundering, even energy efficiency. A division of Google's DeepMind team was able to improve the cooling efficiency at Google's own data centers by more than 40%. Data centers consume about 3% of global energy usage each year—so imagine the impact on the environment if we could apply these systems across the world.[3]

As the barriers to entry go down we will see opportunities for businesses of all kinds to take advantage of what AI can do. The medical field will be transformed by AI. Here are a few examples that are already impacting and changing medical practice. CSAIL's Regina Barzilay has teamed with doctors at Massachusetts General Hospital to use *machine learning* to improve detection and prevent overtreatment in breast cancer.[4] Their method correctly diagnosed 97% of breast cancers as malignant and reduced the number of benign surgeries by more than 30% compared with existing approaches. DeepMind is teaming with doctors to train AI to help plan treatments for cancer. IBM's Watson AI is being trialed by doctors at 55 hospitals around the world because of its success rate at identifying tumors.[5] AI is also enabling the discovery of new treatments. In the past it took around 12 years to get a new drug to market, with a cost of about $2.6 billion. But now *machine learning* algorithms allow computers to "learn" how to choose what experiments need to be done.[6] Recently researchers using this technique announced that they'd already seen promising results in delaying the onset of amyotrophic lateral sclerosis.[7]

It is important to note that AI is not replacing doctors. It can't sit down with patients, discuss their diagnosis, or review treatment plans, but it can help doctors

---

[2] https://hms.harvard.edu/news/better-together.

[3] http://www.wired.co.uk/article/mustafa-suleyman-deepmind-google-ai.

[4] http://news.mit.edu/2017/putting-data-in-the-hands-of-doctors-regina-barzilay-0216.

[5] http://www.bbc.com/fature/story/20170914-spotting-cancer-stopping-shootings-how-ai-protects-us.

[6] https://techcrunch.com/2017/03/16/advances-in-ai-and-ml-are-reshaping-healthcare/.

[7] https://www.usnews.coWnews/technology/articles/2017-08-10/how-ai-robots-hunt-new-drugs-for-crippling-nerve-disease.

make the right diagnoses and recognize all the available treatment options—all while freeing up time to actually spend with their patients.

Such AI advances are great examples of what is known in the computer science literature as "Narrow AI." Current systems are capable of looking at vast amounts of data, extracting patterns, making predictions, and acting based on those predictions. With a game like Go the computer can study every game ever recorded and model every likely outcome. However, if you expanded the board size, the system would have trouble running exhaustive searches due to the exponential growth of the number of options. The Go program also does not know how to play chess, poker, or other games. In contrast, "General AI" refers to a system that demonstrates intelligent behavior as advanced or more advanced than a human across a broad range of cognitive tasks, but this part of AI is decades away. Even with the major advances being made today, AI is nowhere close to people in breadth and depth of human perception, reasoning, communication, and creativity. It can't undertake creative intelligence tasks or put together unfamiliar combinations of ideas. It lacks social intelligence.

While AI has the potential to be a vector for incredible positive change, it is important to understand what today's state of the art is: what today's methods can and cannot do. The intelligence problem—how the brain produces intelligent behavior and how machines can replicate it—remains a profound challenge in science and engineering requiring well-trained researchers and sustained long-term research and innovation to solve.

# Databases

# Machine Learning and Massive Health Data

## Partnership Between the Caisse Nationale d'Assurance Maladie and the École Polytechnique

Emmanuel Bacry and Stéphane Gaïffas

## Introduction

At the end of 2014 the Caisse nationale d'Assurance maladie (CNAM) and the École polytechnique signed a three-year research and development partnership agreement.[1] Extended until the end of 2020 this partnership aims to promote the development of Big Data technologies applied to the health sector. More precisely, this collaboration aims to deploy new ways of exploiting the data of the National Information System Inter Plans Health Insurance (SNIIRAM). This database mainly gathers data on reimbursements and hospitalization of beneficiaries of all compulsory health insurance schemes in France (see C. Gissot's chapter in this book[2]). This is not a clinical database but an Electronic Health Records (EHR) database. These bases are very rich and their analysis has become a subject of study in its own right and the source

---

[1]This partnership is above all a team effort. The results are down to the collaboration of highly multidisciplinary teams. We would like to thank the doctors, developers, researchers, and business experts of CNAM (in particular, Aurélie Bannay, Hélène Caillol, Joël Coste, Claude Gissot, Fanny Leroy, Anke Neumann, Jérémie Rudant, and Alain Weill) and the teams of developers, data scientists, and researchers at the École Polytechnique (in particular, Prosper Burq, Philip Deegan, Nguyen Dinh Phong, Xristos Giastidis, Agathe Guilloux, Daniel de Paula da Silva, Youcef Sebiat, and Dian Sun).

[2]See the chapter titled "Medical and Administrative Data on Health Insurance," p. 75 in this book.

---

E. Bacry (✉)
University of Paris-Dauphine and Ecole Polytechnique, Paris, France
e-mail: bacry@ceremade.dauphine.fr

S. Gaïffas
University of Paris-Diderot, Paris, France

© Springer Nature Switzerland AG 2020
B. Nordlinger et al. (eds.), *Healthcare and Artificial Intelligence*,
https://doi.org/10.1007/978-3-030-32161-1_4

of many research articles.[3] Through SNIIRAM France is fortunate to have one of the largest EHR databases in the world. With more than 65 million health files, 1.2 billion reimbursements per year, and 11 million hospital stays this database weighs more than 200 tonnes. Of incredible richness, its analysis is of the utmost importance both for potential health and economic impacts (the public health budget is the first budget of the French State). CNAM teams of statisticians have been working on this for several years and have obtained many important results such as those obtained in 2013 on the thromboembolic risk of third-generation pills.

The current machine infrastructure, data organization, and software solutions of CNAM were designed to optimize the initial purpose of SNIIRAM (namely, the reimbursement of care), but are not well suited to methodological research. This is a major factor limiting systematic large-scale data mining that is the standard in the world of Big Data and artificial intelligence, exploration of unknown territories, and promising innovation.

This partnership aims to develop algorithms defined with regard to the tasks of CNAM and, more broadly, to public health issues. Disruptive algorithms can be used to detect weak signals or anomalies in pharmacoepidemiology, to identify factors useful for the analysis of care pathways, or to assist in the fight against abuse and fraud. Such developments have necessitated a rethinking of CNAM's infrastructure (i.e., machine infrastructure, data organization, and analysis tools). These are the initial results of the first three years of this unique experience both in terms of the scope of the task and its potential societal impacts that we propose to describe briefly here. This is very largely a collective work benefiting from an exceptional multidisciplinary framework bringing together data scientists, developers, researchers in mathematics or computer science, and SNIIRAM business experts, as well as medical specialists in public health.

## CNAM Infrastructure Revisited

The current CNAM infrastructure is not designed to facilitate large-scale statistical analysis since this is a barrier to methodological research. To successfully carry out our partnership and be able to focus on new approaches it quickly became unavoidable to rid ourselves of the entire data-processing chain (or pipeline). A team of engineers specializing in Big Data technologies have been working on this long-term project, the very first version of which was delivered after two years (this is an ongoing work). The work consisted essentially of three points.

---

[3]Coloma P., "Mining Electronic Healthcare Record Databases to Augment Drug Safety Surveillance," PhD Manuscript, University Medical Center, Rotterdam, 2012; Morel M., Bacry E., Gaïffas S. et al. "ConvSCCS: convolutional self-controlled case series model for lagged adverse event detection," *ArXiv preprint*, 2017; Rajkomar A., Oren E., Chen K. et al. "Scalable and accurate *deep learning* for electronic health records," *ArXiv preprint*, 2018; Shickel B., Tighe P., Bihorac A. et al. "Deep EHR: A Survey of Recent Advances in *Deep Learning* Techniques for Electronic Health Record (EHR) Analysis," *ArXiv e-prints*, 2018.

## From a Vertical to a Horizontal Architecture

As part of the partnership we set up a horizontal machine infrastructure at CNAM that allows distributed computing. It is a standard infrastructure in today's world that splits the enormity of data into several much smaller packages that can be managed by relatively low-cost machines. These slave machines send their results to master machines that compile them and centralize the results of calculations. Scaling is done mainly by adding slave machines where the current infrastructure, centered on high-powered computers (Exadata, manufactured by Oracle) managing very large amounts of data alone (*vertical* architecture), requires very large investments. This new horizontal architecture (combined with the Spark library, another Big Data standard) makes it possible to read *all* the data efficiently and repeatedly, a prerequisite to the entire processing pipeline that we describe below.

## Flattening the Data

The first step in this pipeline involves total reorganization of the data to be able to access them very efficiently. For example, it is necessary to be able to quickly retrieve an insured's entire care history (the insured's data are anonymized: no names, addresses, or social security numbers are accessible). In the current organization the data of a care pathway is broken down into nearly 800 data tables (organized in a proprietary Oracle database) each containing a portion of the pathway. Thus, the central table (of several billion lines for a year of history) lists on each line a particular refund. To access the details of such a refund each line points to the lines of other tables (relational logic) and so on thus connecting the 800 tables. The flattening of these data into the equivalent of a very large table (distributed on slave machines) enables us today to compile very efficiently all types of information (such as a care path).

## Software Development

We carried out a number of computer code developments to flatten the data just mentioned and to develop new machine-learning models. Such developments are essentially of two types.

The development of a library of standardized interfaces enabling access to these data not only at the granular level (reimbursement data), but also at the level of health events (prescriptions for medication, outbreaks of illness, etc.). The aim is to develop a generic grammar to facilitate (for non-specialists) the preparation of raw data into digital data that can be used by machine learning algorithms.

The development of machine learning algorithms in commonly used standard development frameworks (such as R software and Python) without the need for proprietary tools (such as SAS software currently at the center of statistical analysis at CNAM) is highly efficient at traditional statistical analysis, but does not allow algorithmic innovation.

It should be noted that the pipeline described above has not yet been developed for the entire database. It was indeed necessary to quickly carry out a proof of concept on part of this basis. For example, we have not yet used purely accounting data since we have focused exclusively on information describing the health events of the insured. Knowing that all the tools used in this project are standards from the Big Data world scaling becomes a minor problem. Moreover, it is worth noting that they are all free of rights (open source) and so by definition very open to unlimited methodological research. The corresponding open source libraries, referred to as SCALPEL3, are described in reference 12.

## Toward an Automatic Screening Algorithm for Drugs with Harmful Side Effects

Identifying a drug on the market that may cause adverse side effects is a very sensitive issue. The issue is obviously of primary importance, but the side effect (no matter how serious) is never systematic and corresponds to an effect of small magnitude compared with the reported effect of the drug and is therefore very difficult to detect. We are talking about the detection of weak signals. To do this the state of the art in biostatistics is to do hypothesis validation using survival models, the most classical model of which is Cox regression.[4] The various steps of this approach can essentially be broken down into five phases:

1. Choice of a drug $M$ and a specific side effect $E$. The hypothesis that the survival model seeks to validate or invalidate is: "Does a patient's exposure to $M$ increase the risk of $E$?"
2. Definition of exposure by a group of expert doctors. What is the minimum number of doses given patients before they are considered exposed to $M$? Should these dosages be normalized over time?
3. Data on extracting the care pathway of all the insured (called a cohort) who have been exposed to $M$ (as defined above).
4. Homogenizing the cohort (carried out according to rules established by the same experts). For example, the model does not allow putting into the same "basket" someone who developed the $E$ effect one month after exposure to $M$ and someone who developed the same effect two years after exposure.
5. Applying the survival model to the cohort of patients exposed to $M$ should lead to validation of the hypothesis with a certain level of confidence. To do this the

---

[4]Cox D., "Regression Models and Life-Tables," *Journal of the Royal Statistical Society*, Series B. 1972.

model is based on comparing the subcohort of patients who have developed $E$ with the control subcohort of patients who have not developed $E$.

This tried-and-tested process continues to prove its worth. However, it has two major disadvantages: $M$ and $E$ must be defined a priori; and steps 2 and 4 are the result of delicate expert discussions that make the entire process relatively long (it typically takes several months to obtain reliable answers). This makes it totally prohibitive to conduct systematic large-scale analysis on a large number of drugs and/or side effects.

The first three years of work undertaken by the partnership fell within this framework: the development of an algorithm for automatic drug screening that increases the risk of a given side effect, and an algorithm that requires only occasional intervention by experts reducing steps 2 and 4 previously described to their strict minimum. Of course, such an algorithm cannot be expected to be as accurate as a conventional analysis using a survival model specific to a precise torque $(M, E)$. With its unprecedented speed of development, such an algorithm should be considered a preliminary step to identifying those likely to be problematic across a large number of drugs. The drugs identified in this way will require further analysis for confirmation. This screening algorithm therefore intervenes upstream of traditional analyses (survival type) and will enable large-scale rapid screening for the first time.

## ConvSCCS: A Large-Scale Screening Algorithm

The ConvSCCS algorithm is based on the self-controlled case series (SCCS[5]) principle. Only patients who have developed the side effect studied (hence the name "case series" in SCCS) are included in the study. Control is no longer done with a cohort of patients who did not contract the side effect, but with patients who contracted it before the effect appeared. The patient thus plays the role of his/her own control (hence the name "self-controlled" in SCCS): the period when the patient contracts the side effect is implicitly compared with the period when the patient has not yet contracted it although he/she is already exposed to the drugs to be tested. The use of this type of model is an interesting alternative to using Cox's proportional risk model to identify drugs with adverse side effects.

The ConvSCCS algorithm has two main advantages over Cox's proportional risk model. First, it significantly improves the level of the signals to be detected making the signals less weak and therefore easier to detect than with a Cox regression survival model. This is because the number of patients who have developed the side effect is much smaller than the number of patients exposed to the drug under consideration, a problem that disappears when no further subcohort control is considered. Second,

[5]Schuemie M., Trifirò G., Coloma P. et al., "Detecting adverse drug reactions following long-term exposure in longitudinal observational data: The exposure- adjusted self-controlled case series," *Statistical Methods in Medical Research*, 2014; Whitaker H., Paddy Farrington C., Spiessens B. et al., "Tutorial in biostatistics: The self-controlled case series method," *Statistics in Medicine*, 2006.

it significantly reduces the effect of bias potentially present in the data. This type of model is only sensitive to variations in the longitudinal variables considered (values that change over the period of time considered) such as drug exposures. Static variables, such as the patient's gender, do not impact the results of such a model.

However, standard algorithms of the SCCS type are not without defects. Our ConvSCCS[6] algorithm has very significant improvements that are particularly suitable for large-scale automatic screening.

ConvSCCS allows the potential effect of several drugs to be modeled simultaneously, whereas conventional SCCS methods allow only one drug to be studied at a time. ConvSCCS is therefore much less sensitive to the effects of drug confusion. Indeed, a patient is often exposed in his/her care journey to several drugs leading to these exposures sometimes being superimposed. The model tends to confuse the effect of a drug with the effect of those not used in the modeling when not enough drugs are incorporated in the model.

ConvSCCS has good robustness properties that reduce the sensitivity of results obtained by the model to preliminary work of the experts (steps 2 and 4). Steps 2 and 4 can then be reduced to relatively brief work.

ConvSCCS makes it possible to obtain curves quantifying the influence of exposure to each drug as a function of time on the probability of the side effect occurring. This algorithm therefore automatically learns the exposure times that may lead to risk for the side effect occurring, which was not the case with other SCCS methods. To do this we use a technique called penalization that will force the coefficients learned by the model to have a "simple" structure, while explaining the data correctly. In Fig. 1 we observe constant curves per piece over relatively long intervals. This form of curve is precisely the one sought here. We want to detect statistically significant changes in values interpreted as significant changes in the influence of exposure after a certain period of time on the probability of the side effect occurring. In addition, these curves are calculated by gauging the estimation uncertainty of these influences.

## First Results Obtained Using the ConvSCCS Algorithm: Identification of an Antidiabetic Agent Increasing the Risk for Bladder Cancer

The first results obtained with ConvSCCS are related to a pilot project set up by the partnership. The objective was "blind" detection of pioglitazone that has a side effect of bladder cancer overrisk. This was confirmed in a study[7] leading to its withdrawal from the market in 2011. This specific example was chosen in conjunction with

[6]Morel M., Bacry E., Gaïffas S., Gaiffas, A.., Leroy, F. "ConvSCCS: convolutional self-controlled case-series model for lagged adverse event detection". Biostatistics, kxz003, https://doi.org/10.1093/biostatistics/kxz003 (2019).

[7]Neumann A., Weill A., Ricordeau P. et al., "Pioglitazone and risk of bladder cancer among diabetic patients in France: a population-based cohort study," *Diabetologia*, 2012.

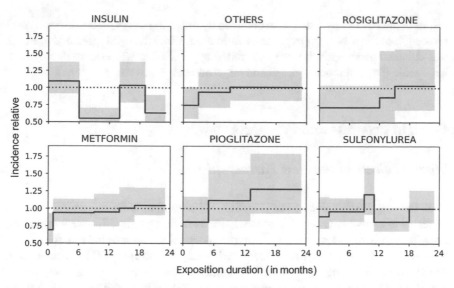

**Fig. 1** Estimates of exposure effects to various antidiabetic drugs on the risk for bladder cancer. We observe that only pioglitazone has an effect significantly greater than 1

CNAM public health physicians because it is considered a weak signal. Pioglitazone has been withdrawn from the market in France,[8] but not everywhere in the world.[9] This pilot project therefore consisted of finding this effect (already known to CNAM) to validate two aspects of our approach: the pipeline (that reshapes all data processing) by precisely reproducing the results obtained in the study using Cox regressions; and the validity of ConvSCCS as an alternative algorithm to blindly find the effect of this molecule by greatly simplifying steps 1 to 5 described earlier. ConvSCCS also brings a large number of improvements as already mentioned.

The study was based on a cohort of 2.5 million patients with a four-year history of type 2 diabetes. The data spread over approximately two billion lines (1.3 TB). The adverse event considered was bladder cancer, and we considered exposures to the antidiabetic drugs listed in Fig. 1. On this dataset the steps of flattening and preparing the data required about 40 min of calculation. Training the model (machine learning phase) took only a few minutes (done with our tick[10] library). We illustrate in Fig. 1 the curves obtained by the model. These curves quantify the impact of exposures to antidiabetic molecules over time on bladder cancer risk. Value 1 corresponds to an absence of effect (in both directions). Around this value the molecule has no impact on risk. It can be seen that only pioglitazone has an effect significantly greater than 1, and this after an exposure of just over a year. This result was fully consistent with the

---

[8]Ibid.

[9]Lewis J., Habel L., Quesenberry C. et al., "Pioglitazone use and risk of bladder cancer and other common cancers in persons with diabetes," *JAMA*, 2015.

results of the 2012 study[10] that were obtained by following a very precise biostatistical protocol (see steps 1–5) for hypothesis validation, while the result obtained in Fig. 1 was obtained using a much more automated approach that was easy to deploy on a large scale (large number of drugs and large number of adverse reactions).

## Work in Progress and Prospects

### *Study Projects of the New Partnership*

Even the very first version of the ConvSCCS[11] algorithm is mature enough now to be tested in a "real situation." That is what we are doing today. We are working on drugs currently on the market that have the potential to increase the risk for falls in the elderly. CNAM experts have identified nearly 250 drugs (150 molecules) that need to be studied ranging from antihypertensives, antidepressants, neuroleptics, to hypnotics. The cohort we are interested in contains nearly 12 million people whose data spread over about 2 billion lines per year. Flattening and data preparation take less than two hours and model training takes as always only a few minutes.

This is achieved by genuinely scaling up (by a factor of about 4) the diabetes pilot project. Scaling up the entire pipeline not only including machine and software infrastructure but also the algorithm itself supports a greater quantity of data and robustness in relation to this change of problem. Indeed, the pilot project concerns long-term effects (at least one year of waiting before seeing the effect of pioglitazone exposure), while in the case of falls the effect if any is short term (a few days). We are also working on other important improvements including the possibility of simultaneously taking into account several side effects, or even automatically detecting what the side effects of a particular drug are.

In parallel with this pharmacovigilance research work and its effective implementation two other themes are being addressed by the partnership: the fight against fraud and the identification of factors useful for the analysis of care pathways. We have begun an interactive visualization process of a large number of care pathways, an essential step in understanding the pathways within a given pathology. We are also working on other machine learning techniques including *deep learning* and artificial intelligence techniques.

---

[10]Bacry E., Bompaire M., Gaïffas S. et al., "Tick: A Python library for statistical learning, with a particular emphasis on time-dependent modeling," *Journal of Machine Learning Research*, 2018.

[11]Morel M., Bacry E., Gaïffas S. et al., 2017, art. cit. 12 "SCALPEL3 : a scalable open-source library for healthcare claims databases", *Arxiv preprint (arXiv:1910.07045)*, 2019.

## Toward Systematizing and Opening up the Big Data Pipeline

All the developments that have been made within the framework of the partnership have been made so that they can be used by non-Big Data experts. Transfer of knowledge has already begun *by* pooling IT developers. Our ambition is for our Big Data pipeline to be a proof of concept for larger scale opening up of the pipeline (all the software we have developed is free of rights), an alternative pipeline to the one currently present in SNDS that defines the legal framework for access to SNIIRAM. Our Big Data pipeline can also be used as proof of concept for the Health Data Hub announced by the President of France when the Villani Report was submitted on March 29, 2018. This dataset is unique in the world and the source of so much wealth, yet it is still largely underexploited for the common good.

# Linking an Epidemiological Cohort to Medicoadministrative Databases

## Experience of Constances

Marie Zins and Marcel Goldberg

## Cohort Complementarity and Medicoadministrative Databases

The study of health at the population level is currently undergoing profound changes due to the combination of several phenomena: the availability of medico-administrative databases covering entire populations; the establishment of very large epidemiological cohorts in the general population; and the development of new analytical methods based on artificial intelligence. In the following we will present the experience of Constances, a large epidemiological cohort in the general population linked to two national databases covering almost the entire French population: the National Health Data System (NHDS) and the databases of the "Caisse nationale d'assurance vieillesse" (CNAV). Each of these databases s a very rich source of individual data but has limitations that can be partially overstated by pooling them.[1] However, for this potential to be realized and fully exploited many scientific, methodological, and technical difficulties must be overcome.

---

[1]The Constances cohort is funded by the ANR (ANR-11-INBS-0002).

---

M. Zins (✉) · M. Goldberg
University of Paris Descartes and INSERM, Paris, France
e-mail: marie.zins@inserm.fr

M. Goldberg
e-mail: marcel.goldberg@inserm.fr

© Springer Nature Switzerland AG 2020
B. Nordlinger et al. (eds.), *Healthcare and Artificial Intelligence*,
https://doi.org/10.1007/978-3-030-32161-1_5

## National Health Data System

France is one of the few countries to have centralized national medicosocial and socioeconomic databases built and managed by public bodies exhaustively and permanently covering the entire population. In addition, a unique individual identifier (the French social security number or NIR) is currently being used (directly or in encrypted form) by practically all national databases whose creation is based on activities related to the tasks of the administration and public bodies. A major interest is that they are exhaustive and regularly produced. The use of these databases offers very important advantages both in methodological (exhaustiveness, absence of selection and information biases) and operational (data already collected, huge numbers of subjects, etc.) terms. They obviously have various limitations in terms of data coverage, quality, and validity that vary according to the types of use that can be envisaged. These databases concerning more than 60 million people nevertheless constitute a considerable intangible heritage probably unparalleled in the world in terms of their exhaustiveness, richness, and size of the population covered. We will only deal here with the NHDS.

The data produced by the operation of health insurance and hospital systems are collected in the National Information System Inter Plans Health Insurance (SNIIRAM), the main component of the NHDS managed by CNAM.[2]

SNIIRAM combines two data sources. The Medicalization of In-training Systems Program (PMSI) allows the exhaustive collection of administrative and medical information for each hospital stay including diagnoses coded according to the International Classification of Diseases (ICD-10) and procedures performed according to the Common Classification of Medical Procedures (CCAM). The DCIR database (interscheme care consumption data) includes health insurance data such as ambulatory care (consultations, medical procedures, biology, medical devices, medicines), eligible conditions (long-term conditions, ALD), disabilities, accidents at work, and occupational diseases coded in ICD-10. Since 2014 causes of death have also been included in the NHDS.

SNIIRAM is an individual database where all information about the same person is linked using a unique identifier. To this end patients' NIRs are irreversibly encrypted before being integrated into SNIIRAM thanks to the FOIN (nominal information occlusion function) hash module that produces an anonymous, non-reversible identifier. From an identifier the nominal data used to calculate it cannot be found. It is important to note that calculation of this identifier is based on the NIR, which means that to find a person's data in SNIIRAM it is necessary to have her/his NIR. Similarly, when you wish to access the individual data contained in SNIIRAM (e.g., to link

---

[2]Tuppin P., Rudant J., Constantinou P., Gastaldi-Ménager C., Rachas A., de Roquefeuil L., Maura G., Stone H., Tajahmady A., Coste J., Gissot C., Weill A., Fagot-Campagna A., "Value of a national administrative database to guide public decisions: From the national interregime information system of l'Assurance maladie (SNIIRAM) to the système national des données de santé (SNDS) in France," *Rev Epidemiol Sante Publique*, October 2017, 65, suppl. 4, S149–S167.

cohort data with SNIIRAM data), you must obtain the NIR of the persons concerned to be able to calculate their SNIIRAM identifier by the FOIN procedure.

Article 193 of the recent law for the modernization of the French health system has greatly simplified the possibilities of accessing NHDS data, and it is expected that requests for access to this exceptional database will increase rapidly once the new legal and organizational framework is in place.

However, it is not an exaggeration to say that once access to SNIIRAM has been obtained the real difficulties begin. These difficulties are due in large part to the fact that this is a gigantic and highly complex database that concerns three main aspects: volume, data architecture, and data interpretation. This is because SNIIRAM consists of production data intended for the control and reimbursement of health services that require very good knowledge of the regulatory and technical context of reimbursement to be used correctly.

In terms of volume 1.2 billion care sheets are transferred each year from SNIIRAM and 1000 flows are received each month from data-processing centers, other schemes, mutuals, regional health insurance funds, etc. A total of nearly 20 billion service lines are available. There are 17 databases 3 of which have a volume of more than 25 TB. A total of 150 applications are managed with a storage capacity of 450 TB.

In terms of architecture SNIIRAM has 7 dictionaries with 785,000 objects (tables, indexes, synonyms, etc.). The care consumption part of SNIIRAM has 12 tables and about 300 variables. In addition, the number of tables and variables change each year in the PMSI part of SNIIRAM. To construct a "useful" variable it is necessary to join several tables. All information about a person in the DCIR part of SNIIRAM is focused on the benefits reimbursed. A set of tables more precisely characterizing the elements of these services is therefore attached to a central "Services" table. On average, there are several dozen lines per person in the central Services table, some of which are "polluting" data purely intended for reimbursement and invoicing (lines used to cancel a reimbursement, surcharges, flat rate contributions, deductibles, etc.) that make it necessary to clean up the data so that only information relevant to the user is kept.

When it comes to making sense of the data many aspects must be known before making a request and analyzing the results. Knowledge of the nomenclatures used is indispensable such as the precise nature of the treatments, procedures, and examinations corresponding to the pathology of interest. For example, to identify women who have had a cervical smear in the last three years it should be noted that recent years have given rise to three different codifications due to changes in regulations. To find all patients who have had a cervical smear over the last three years a total of five tables have to be investigated (plus another two for identifiers) with three different joint keys and in two environments (PMSI/DCIR).

It is also necessary to be aware of invoicing methods (acts and services included in hospital stays invoiced in addition to fixed prices, retroceded, carried out in day hospitals and/or in full hospitalization); different invoicing in the private and public sectors; local specificities (DOM, Alsace Moselle regime); modalities related to the social characteristics of individuals (universal health coverage, CMU); complementary universal health coverage (CMU-C) and State medical aid (AME) sometimes different from the general regime (MSA, RSI); and delays in data transmission by institutions and professionals sometimes not homogeneous throughout the territory. In addition, answers to these questions are constantly evolving in response to rapidly changing regulations.

The data extracted from SNIIRAM by CNAM are most often provided to the user in raw form, and it is up to the user to synthesize this information to obtain the constructed variables that really are of interest. To make the SNIIRAM enlargement usable a significant amount of methodological and technical work is therefore required.

In short, the NHDS is clearly of major interest in that it provides individual medicalized, structured, and standard coded data for the entire population. However, in addition to the difficulties listed it has certain limitations in terms of recorded data: absence of data on risk factors associated with diseases, virtual absence of data on socioprofessional status, no clinical or paraclinical examination results, validity of health data of variable quality that may require significant control and validation work.

For all these reasons optimal use of the exceptional potential of the NHDS requires the development of complementary approaches such as linking individual data sources including epidemiological cohorts and developing tools to facilitate data understanding and manipulation.


# The Constances Cohort

The objective of Constances[3] is to implement a large epidemiological cohort to provide information for public health purposes and to contribute to the development of health research. Led by the Population Epidemiological Cohorts unit (Inserm UMS 011), in partnership with CNAM and the Caisse nationale d'assurance vieillesse (CNAV), the Constances Cohort (Infrastructure nationale en biologie et santé—part of the Investments d'avenir) aims to build an infrastructure that is widely accessible to the public health and epidemiological research community.

Constances consists of a random sample of the population covered by the General Social Security Scheme between the ages of 18 and 69.[4] Total population size is 200,000 structured to be proportional to the population for gender, age, and social category. Eligible persons are those living in the 21 French departments whose Health Examination Centers (HECs) participate in Constances (Fig. 1).

Once included in the cohort volunteers benefiting from a complete health examination in their CES are then asked to complete questionnaires relating to health, lifestyle, professional history, occupational exposure, etc. Moreover, blood and urine samples are taken to establish a biobank.

---

[3] www.constances.fr.

[4] Zins M, Goldberg M, the Constances team, "The French CONSTANCES population-based cohort: Design, inclusion and follow-up," *Eur J Epidemiology*, 2015, 30, 1317–1328.

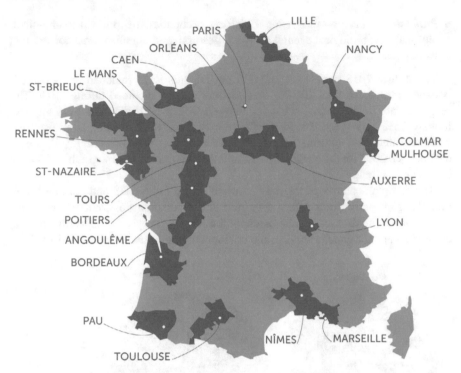

**Fig. 1** Geographical distribution of Health Examination Centers participating in Constances

Volunteer follow-up is twofold: active by questionnaire each year and invitation to return to the CES every four years for a new health examination; passive by linkage to the NHDS (health and care use data) and CNAV databases (socioprofessional events).

From inception and during follow-up a lot of data are collected:

- *Health data*—personal and family history; self-reported health and quality-of-life scales; reported pathologies, long-term illness and hospitalizations; absences from work; disabilities, limitations, and trauma; medical cause of death; health behaviors (tobacco, alcohol, food, physical activity, cannabis, sexual orientation); female-specific health problems.
- *Use of care and management*—health professionals; medicines; medical devices; biology; ALD; PMSI.
- *Health examination*—weight, height, waist–hip ratio, blood pressure, electrocardiogram, vision, hearing, spirometry, biological investigations. People aged 45 and over are given tests to assess physical and cognitive functional abilities. Biological samples are stored in a biobank.
- *Sociodemographic characteristics*—occupational status and activity; level of education; income level; marital status; household composition; socioeconomic status of parents and spouse; material living conditions.

• *Professional factors*—professional history; occupational exposures to chemical, physical, and biological agents; postural, gestural, and organizational constraints; work stress.

As of July 2018 more than 180,000 participants were included. Moreover, it is expected that the final 200,000 participants will be included during 2019. The response rate to the annual self-administered follow-up questionnaire is approximately 75% each year. The data obtained by linkage to medico-administrative databases include all information since CNAV databases were first employed, and all events since 2009 for the NHDS. The sample has a good sociodemographic diversity as shown in Fig. 2.

The complementarity of the data extracted from the NHDS and data collected directly from participants offers very rich and diversified possibilities for analysis in various fields such as pharmacoepidemiology, analyses of care trajectories, etiological and prognostic studies, and socioeconomic impact studies of diseases.

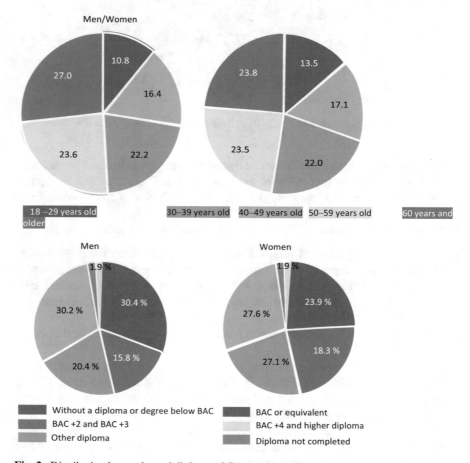

**Fig. 2** Distribution by gender and diploma of Constances participants

## Tools to Help Understand and Manipulate Data

Due to the complexity of the SNIIRAM database the team in charge of Constances had to develop a series of tools to make optimal use of the data from this source. Examples of these tools are briefly described here, but there are many other developments that are equally desirable.

### Interactive Documentation

Due to the complexity and scalability of the data that make up SNIIRAM it is essential to have the most complete and up-to-date documentation possible for each information domain (DCIR, PMSI–MCO, etc.) to understand data specifications, management rules, nomenclatures used, etc. To this end interactive documentation of SNIIRAM data has been developed to include several particulars such as generalities, presentation of the domains covered (DCIR, PMSI–MCO, PMSI–SSR, etc.), description of the data (presentation of tables and variables, specific information on variables, etc.), health insurance concepts and useful definitions, nomenclatures, and value tables. In addition, documentary monitoring is necessary due to SNIIRAM constantly evolving: addition or disappearance of tables, variables, modification of the institutional perimeter (general regime, SLM, RSI, MSA, etc.), modification of management rules, modification of nomenclatures, etc.

### Receipt of SNIIRAM Data

Constances is matched to SNIIRAM once a year. The first task to be done before you can work on the the data provided by CNAM consists in verifying that the data correspond to the request since there may be problems during the extraction and transmission of these files. When sending SNIIRAM data CNAM requests collecting the data and returning the data within three months. Due to the complexity and volume of data manual verification is particularly cumbersome and tedious. This has led to develop a specific software to facilitate verification of the data received. This involves several control steps that correspond to the various types of errors that may occur when extracting SNIIRAM data such as absence of requested tables, empty tables and variables, data format (name, size), and inconsistency of file lines. Once data integration has been completed postintegration checks are systematically carried out. They cover identifiers, all dates, variables of joins between tables and certain variables of interest (nature of reference service, exemption from user fees on medicalized tables, etc.).

## Construction of Calculated Data

Due to the difficulties described above raw SNIIRAM data must be preprocessed to construct the variables that need to be integrated into the cohort databases for use. Depending on what is required various approaches are implemented:

- *Construction of dummy variables*—these are binary or numerical variables (counts) used to indicate the occurrence of an event or a number of events over a period for a subject in the Constances database. These variables relate to the scope of the data (presence in the DCIR, presence in the PMSI–MCO, etc.) or to a characteristic of a subject such as care consumption and hospitalization data (procedures, diagnoses, homogeneous groups of patients, additional drugs, etc.). This construction requires a number of steps such as checking whether documentation on the event in question matches the raw SNIIRAM data based on the interactive documentation already described, the format of the raw data used to check consistency between the specificities described in the documentation and the reality of the SNIIRAM data because the data are not always in line with SNIIRAM management and coding rules.
- *Construction of* ad hoc *indicators*—when questions defined a priori need to be studied work must be tailored to construct the relevant variables by "translating" the requests into SNIIRAM data. A good example concerns the measurement of access to care for people with depression.[5] Relevant data here relate to consultation of a general practitioner within 12 months, the consultation of a psychiatrist within 12 months, and the taking of psychotropic drugs within 12 months (antidepressants, anxiolytics). To construct the relevant variables it is necessary to precisely define the variables of interest by flagging up at least one reimbursement for a consultation or a number of consultations, an annual indicator or indicators constructed from the date of inclusion in the cohort (within 12 months of inclusion), and only consultations or consultations and visits. The same questions arise when receiving psychotropic treatment within 12 months. Once again the variables of interest should be defined by flagging up the number of boxes, the number of deliveries, an annual indicator or from the date of inclusion in the Constances Cohort (within 12 months of inclusion), and the CIP or ATC codes used (three or seven characters). This work is particularly time-consuming and requires very good knowledge of the database and a good understanding of the questions asked.
- *Construction of simplified tables from SNIIRAM*—in some cases it is a question of working on variables not identified in advance such as studying multimedication in diabetic patients or those over 45 years of age, concomitant/cumulative use of anticholinergic drugs, and impact on cognitive functions. In these examples we may have to take into account hundreds of drugs some of which do not correspond to official indications of the pathologies concerned. Other examples concern the

---

[5]Melchior M., Ziad A., Courtin E., Zins M., van der Waerden J., "Intergenerational socioeconomic mobility and adult depression: The CONSTANCES study," *Am J Epidemiol.*, 2018, février; 187(2), pp. 260–269.

analysis of time-critical care trajectories such as therapeutic escalation in diabetic patients, strategy after failure of the first line in antidepressant treatment, and identification of the misuse of medicines. In all these cases the construction of ad hoc indicators is neither relevant nor feasible. The solution lies in simplified database in which the main care events (present in SNIIRAM) for each subject are included in the study in one line such as purchases of drugs, consultations, medical biology procedures, hospitalizations, and ALDs. This restructuring of SNIIRAM data facilitates the implementation of Big Data analysis methods such as clustering, visualization, and manipulation and visualization of trajectories.

## The REDSIAM Network

In addition to the tools it develops for its own needs UMS 011 also participates in the REDSIAM[6] network, which it coordinates under the aegis of the main SNIIRAM[7] data producers and users. The interest in REDSIAM is due to the fact that medicalized data from DCIR and PMSI cannot be considered exhaustive in isolation and are not validated according to the usual epidemiological criteria; moreover, the codes used for diagnoses and procedures may vary according to the source, be imprecise, or even incorrect. In short, the use of PMSI as a source of information on diseases is delicate and diagnoses are not always reliable, ALDs have known limits, and the health insurance reimbursement database does not include direct information on the nature of the diseases treated. It is therefore essential to use specific pathology algorithms based on combinations of PMSI diagnostics, ALD, data on medical technical procedures, consumption of drugs or other health products more or less specific to the pathology concerned, consultations with professionals, etc. REDSIAM, which brings together many teams working on SNIIRAM data, aims to carry out methodological work to develop, evaluate, and make available such algorithms by sharing experiences, and sharing and capitalizing on knowledge.

## Resources Needed for Optimal Use of NHDS Data and Linked Cohorts

The increasing use of the NHDS and the existence of very large cohorts pose new challenges in terms of the resources available to make the most of these immense data sources.

---

[6]www.redsiam.fr/.

[7]Goldberg M., Carton M., Doussin A., Fagot-Campagna A., Heyndrickx E., LeMaitre M., Nicolau J., Quantin C., "The REDSIAM network," *Rev Epidemiol Sante Publique*, October 2017, 65, suppl. 4, S144–S148.

## Computer Resources and Organizational Aspects

The volume and complexity of data require significant, if not very significant, computer storage and computing resources when using Big Data and AI methods to cover large areas. In addition, the NHDS security framework and the implementation of the General Data Protection Regulations (GDPR) impose very strong confidentiality and security constraints that, while justified by the sensitivity of health data and the very high possible impact on the privacy of individuals in the event of misuse, nevertheless require devices for accessing and using these data that far exceed the resources currently available to most potential users.

## Diversified Skills

- *SNIIRAM is a database*—this requires information specialists and database managers.
- *SNIIRAM is a medical database*—the data represent very technical medical and paramedical information requiring a good knowledge of medical and medico-technical procedures, medicines, circumstances of care, therapeutic indications, pathologies, etc. This requires doctors, pharmacists, dentists, nurses, and paramedics.
- *SNIIRAM is a medicoadministrative database*—the data recorded produced within a management framework require a good knowledge of the organization of the healthcare system, social protection, reimbursement and management rules, etc. This requires public health professionals, health insurance managers, hospitals managers, etc.
- *SNIIRAM is a medicoadministrative database established for management purposes and not for research purposes*—knowing the limitations of the data in relation to issues of interest is essential, as is also the case for matched cohort data. This requires epidemiologists, health economists, statisticians, etc.

## Conclusion

The immense prospects opened up (particularly, in the field of artificial intelligence) by the increased availability of very large datasets will require major investments to provide adequate IT resources under satisfactory security conditions, to set up pluridisciplinary teams, and to train data scientists. A huge construction site is now open.

# Medical and Administrative Data on Health Insurance

## CNAM Uses

Claude Gissot

The accumulation of data through the digitalization of processes in the health sector as in other fields has become a challenge for all actors in the sector including health insurance. The issue on healthcare system regulation has resulted as is often the case in the production of dashboards/statistics that are highly oriented toward resource management (monitoring of expenditure and the number of patients benefiting from care). However, these data were often measured at highly decentralized levels (primary fund, hospitals) and national consolidation most often resulted in richness being lost from the basic data. The 1990s and 2000s saw the emergence of comprehensive data sources as the description of inpatient care "Programme de médicalisation des système d'information (PMSI) and the outpatient care data Système d'information inter régimes d'assurance maladie (SNIIRAM), the latter having integrated the relationship with PMSI since its inception in the mid-2000s.

Over the past 15 years CNAM has developed SNIIRAM data use for its own purposes and has shown the value of these data beyond statistics about the amounts reimbursed by health primary insurance.

## What Data Are We Talking About?

The information contained in SNIIRAM is mainly derived from processes involved in care reimbursement such as the reimbursement of claims from primary health insurance funds and the description of hospital stays for PMSI. The advantage of these data lies in the exhaustivity of the care activities and population covered and precise descriptions of the care production activity necessary for reimbursement. They are the result of classifications of procedures or products whose accuracy has greatly increased in the last 20 years. Although the detailed drug code (CIP code) has

C. Gissot (✉)
Caisse Nationale d'Assurance Maladie (National Health Insurance), Paris, France
e-mail: claude.gissot@cnamts.fr

© Springer Nature Switzerland AG 2020
B. Nordlinger et al. (eds.), *Healthcare and Artificial Intelligence*,
https://doi.org/10.1007/978-3-030-32161-1_6

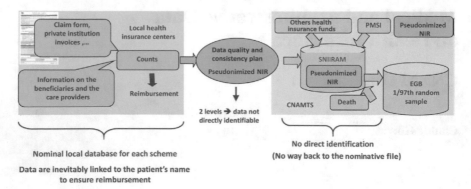

**Fig. 1** SNIIRAM/SNDS collection device. *CNAM*, Caisse nationale de l'Assurance maladie; *EGB echantillon généraliste de bénéficiaires (sample 1% population used for longitudinal studies), NIR,* French social security number; *PMSI,* Programme de médicalisation des systèmes d'information

long been available, the implementation of the common nomenclature of tariff-based medical procedures in the mid-2000s has increased the analytical capabilities of the healthcare system. Other elements that contributed to data enrichment were date of death and detailed coding of the biology.

Another major point the protection of personal data is done by substituting patient identity with a pseudonym that is constant over time and identical in the various databases available such as PMSI and SNIIRAM. Cause of death completes the existing PMSI and SNIIRAM databases both of which are part of the National Health Data System (SNDS). Hence it is possible to link outpatient and inpatient care data and to conduct longitudinal studies on the same individuals over periods of several years.

The data are supplemented in the SNDS by cause of death (2018), data from the medicosocial sector, and a sample of supplementary health insurance reimbursements (Fig. 1).

## CNAM Uses: Management of Disease Risk

The analyses carried out by CNAM cover various aspects of healthcare management such as efficiency of the healthcare system, quality of care and management, support for professionals and institutions, monitoring of healthcare consumption, proper use of care/drugs, pharmacovigilance, and fraud control and enforcement activities. The epidemiology of pathologies treated is another approach that is possible. For a number of years these data were not considered sufficiently precise or of high enough quality to be reused for purposes other than those of initial repayments.

By publishing their studies in high-level journals CNAM demonstrated that these medicoadministrative data have improved sufficiently in quality that they are now capable of providing solid diagnoses on various disorders/illnesses. Publishing the studies has led to health agencies, public and private research operators, and industrialists taking a keen interest in SNIIRAM.

## Analysis of the Healthcare System (Analysis by Provider Moved to Analysis by Disease)

The framework in which expenditure is analyzed (and, more broadly, the health system) is historically linked to regulation such as type of care provider, category of health professional (doctors, pharmacists, nurses, physiotherapist masseur, etc.), and type of hospital. CNAM has developed a tool for medicalized expenditure analysis that makes it possible to reverse the way in which resources are allocated for care. CNAM no longer has a standard analysis by care provider, but instead has a standard analysis by pathology.[1]

Each pathology for which the patient receiving care is treated is defined using algorithms that use all the data available in SNIIRAM. These are deterministic algorithms that cross-reference various information on the reasons for hospital stays, drugs that track pathologies, and medical reasons for copayment exemption from user fees for long-term chronic disease.

These algorithms were compared with different sources that provide information on pathologies and discussed with groups of experts to improve and validate them.

At the same time, cost per item (drugs, generalist/specialist medical fees, etc.) can be established for each person. A method of allocating expenses based on the profiles of population groups with the same pathologies provides a breakdown of costs for each (Fig. 2).

## Care Pathway Studies and Heterogeneity in Care Provision

SNIIRAM contains precise dates of detailed services provided by health professionals and hospitals making it possible to analyze the sequence and care pathway over time. In this way CNAM is able to produce analyses on the heterogeneity of care and the gap between theoretical or standard care pathways and those actually carried out.

Health insurance providers produce annual reports known as "Charges et Produits" that present analyses of various care pathways. Extending beyond their interest in terms of knowledge these analyses are essential inputs into CNAM's efforts to improve efficiency and quality.

---

[1]See chapter "Artificial Intelligence and Tomorrow's Health" in *Health Insurance Annual Proposal Reports*: www.ameli.fr/l-assurance-maladie/statistiques-et-publications/rapports-et-periodicreports/reports-charges-products-of-medical-insurance/index.php.

Numbers by disease (2017- 57,6 millions beneficiaries (General Scheme))

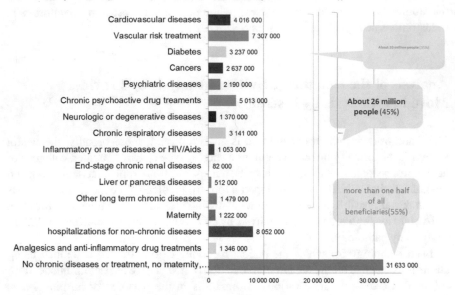

Health expenditure by disease (2017- 140 billions € general scheme - in brackets extent all schemes)

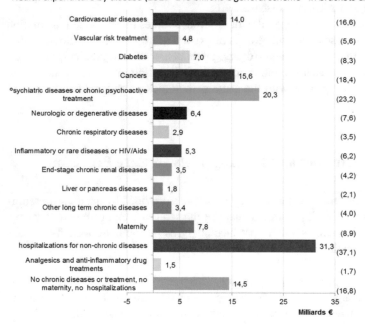

**Fig. 2** Weight of pathologies in terms of number of patients treated and health insurance expenditures

Among the pathways we can find bariatric surgery, EHPAD (institution for elderly people) and antibiotics, cerebrovascular accidents, chronic renal failure, readmissions after a crash to investigate possible bone fragility, etc.

Let us take a detailed look at the pathway of thyroidectomies.

Approximately 40,000 thyroidectomies are performed each year in France. This principally occurs when cancer is suspected following dubious results (low but not zero probability of cancer) from a preoperative puncture. The increase in the frequency of these cancers over the past 20 years (+6% per year) is partly due to a growing trend toward ultrasound screening of nodules leading to an increase in thyroid ablation including for small cancers with a good prognosis. The procedure must be systematically preceded by cytopunction (cell sampling) in the event of a nodule to specify the risk for cancer. According to recommendations of the High Authority for Health, intervention is not justified in the case of a benign nodule. For very small cancers the procedure is very controversial (especially, since it is not trivial and may require lifetime treatment with thyroid hormones, which has its own complications).

Analysis of the care pathway before thyroid ablation surgery shows that necessary procedures are not performed with 18% of patients not having an ultrasound and 69% not having cytopunction, whereas these two procedures should be systematically used. Moreover, scintigraphy is performed in 21% of cases although it is of little use in most cases. Hormonal dosages are not always appropriate. The study concludes that "more than two thirds do not have a quality course, while nearly one in two patients consulted an endocrinologist in the course of the year."

## Real-Life Drug Studies

Several years ago the National Agency for Drug Safety collaborated with CNAM to support the development of skills in the use of data and to build a work program for studies on drugs and their real-life uses. Indeed, real-life drug use analyses are an essential complement to clinical trials.

A few emblematic examples from recent years illustrate this use, which is likely to develop because new drugs are quickly put on the market to take advantage of their innovative nature. However, there needs to be a means of monitoring them to assess their impact under real conditions of use. A good example is bladder cancer risk in diabetics treated with pioglitazone in France (a cohort study using SNIIRAM and PMSI[2] data). In another example CNAM and ANSM conducted a study on the risk of autoimmune disease with HPV vaccination (a report on this was published in the context of questions being asked about the necessity of this vaccination). It has

---

[2] Work carried out by Caisse nationale de l'Assurance maladie des travailleurs salariés (CNAMTS) led to suspension of the use of the antidiabetic pioglitazone in France on June 9, 2011 and its withdrawal from the French market by the Agence du medicament (Afssaps) of pioglitazone (Actos and Competact). Neumann A., Weill A., Ricordeau P., Fagot J.-P., Alla F., Allemand H., "Pioglitazone and risk of bladder cancer among diabetic patients in France: A population-based cohort study," *Diabetologia*, July 2012, 55(7), 1953–1962.

shown reassuring results in terms of the health safety of HPV vaccines, but with a probable increase in the risk of Guillain–Barré syndrome (1 or 2 cases per 100,000 girls vaccinated), which calls into question the balance of benefits and risks of the vaccines concerned.

## From SNIIRAM to NSDS: Developing the Use of Health Data

The reason SNIIRAM (created in 1999) has made all these uses possible is because new data are constantly being made available such as date of death. Data enrichment will continue within the national health data system with cause of death appearing in 2018 followed in the coming years by data provided by departmental disability centers and then sample data from supplementary insurers. Much like SNIIRAM's task, the NSDS provides data that contribute to information on health and the provision of care; medicosocial care and its quality; the definition, implementation, and evaluation of health and social protection policies; knowledge of health expenditure; health insurance expenditure and medicosocial expenditure; information for health or medicosocial professionals; structures and institutions on their activity; surveillance, health monitoring, and safety; research, studies, evaluation, and innovation in the fields of health and medicosocial care.

Access and usage rules have also evolved to make access run more smoothly and faster while at the same time ensuring the security of personal data. Personal data may be used with the authorization of the Commission nationale de l'Informatique et des Libertés (CNIL) on a project by project basis for research, study, and evaluation purposes of public interest in the health sector, or with permanent authorization by decree in the Conseil d'État for state agencies after consulting the CNIL. The purposes behind promoting health products and modifying individual supplementary insurance contracts are explicitly excluded.

Interest in the NSDS lies in its matching potential facilitated by use of pseudonymized NIRs (French social security numbers). However, use of such matches will remain supervised by the CNIL and will no longer require a decree by the Conseil d'État.

## Conclusion

Medicoadministrative data have proven their usefulness as a result of uses developed by CNAM for its own analytical needs. This includes studying care pathways and professional practices to initiate actions to support professionals and patients with the aim of improving the quality of care and thus the efficiency of health insurance expenditure. Such uses have also been developed in recent years in the various health agencies and among researchers. This increase in use will be reinforced in the coming years by NSDS data and by the possibilities of matching with other sources multiplying to such an extent that medical and administrative data will complement data on clinical results.[3]

---

[3]Tuppin P., Rudant J., Constantinou P., Gastaldi-Ménager C., Rachas A., de Roquefeuil L., Maura G., Caillol H., Tajahmady A., Coste J., Gissot C., Weill A., Fagot-Campagna A., Direction de la stratégie des études et des statistiques (DSES), Caisse nationale d'Assurance maladie des travailleurs salariés, "L'utilité d'une base médico-administrative nationale pour guider la décision publique: du système national d'information interrégimes de l'Assurance maladie (SNIIRAM) vers le système national des données de santé (SNDS) en France," October 2017, 65, supplement 4, S149–S167.

# How the SNIIRAM–PMSI Database Enables the Study of Surgical Practices

## Strengths and Limitations

Bertrand Lukacs

## Importance of Cohort Follow-up of Patients Treated in Routine Practice

Medical progress is based in part on the results of client-controlled studies, the best model of which is a double-blind randomized study testing a new treatment compared with a treatment with already-known effects or with a placebo.

These studies are absolutely essential, but they are not sufficient because they have several limitations. They are designed to answer a specific question and only one: You only look for what you want to find. To allow randomization they require patients to be selected according to very specific criteria. This explains why the patients included in these studies are not representative of the patients treated in daily practice. The duration of these studies is often short and does not allow for long-term follow-up of the care pathway.

The interest in cohort follow-up of patients treated in current practice partly fills these limitations. This explains the major interest in this type of analysis in complementarity with "evidence-based medicine" studies to enrich knowledge of the efficiency of a treatment and to understand the care path of patients treated in current practice.

## About Observapur

The Observapur database was created in 2006. This database includes all men treated in France since January 1, 2004 either for a urinary disorder related to a prostate adenoma or for prostate cancer. It consists of the chaining by patient of all the data from

B. Lukacs (✉)
MGH, Paris, France
e-mail: bertrand.lukacs@gmail.com

© Springer Nature Switzerland AG 2020
B. Nordlinger et al. (eds.), *Healthcare and Artificial Intelligence*,
https://doi.org/10.1007/978-3-030-32161-1_7

PMSI (coding of hospitalizations) and SNIIRAM (coding of benefits reimbursed by health insurance).

These two pathologies were chosen because they meet three important criteria that suggest that analyses and interpretations from the SNIIRAM–PMSI database will be relevant and unambiguous. First, they are very common. About 350,000 men are treated each year for mictional disorders related to prostate adenoma, and prostate cancer is the first cancer by frequency in men. Then, the medical treatments of these two pathologies are specific to them since the taking of these drugs indicates the existence of an active disease. Finally, surgical treatments are also specific to these pathologies. This database is probably the oldest SNIIRAM–PMSI database in all disciplines today. Over the past year and a half it has been merged with the Causes of Death Statistics Data (DCFD) and is known as the National Health Data System (NSDS).

## *The Main Lessons Learned*

Our experience has taught us a number of lessons.

Patient-by-patient chaining of PMSI data, all coding for hospitalizations both public and private, and SNIIRAM data covering all services reimbursed by health insurance provide a very good overview of a patient's care path over time regardless of the method of care. When we started this work this point was contested by many.

The analysis of these two populations of patients treated in everyday life confirms that their profiles are very different from those that are selected for inclusion in conventional clinical research studies. They are much more polymeric, which poses the problem of the interaction between all these molecules (Fig. 1).

Such analysis of the care pathway makes it possible to highlight the significant heterogeneity of practice from one region to another, all other things being equal (Fig. 2).

- Analysis of more than 2,000,000 patients.
- Median age of patients: 65 years.
- Many patients are carriers of co-morbidities.
  - Median number of associated chronic treatments:
    five other treatments
    - 25% of patients take
    more than eight other treatments

These co-morbidities are never taken into account in randomized studies, which select patients on restrictive criteria.

Interactions between drugs used by patients in everyday practice are therefore never studied.

**Fig. 1** Observapur: treatments associated with human urinary disorders

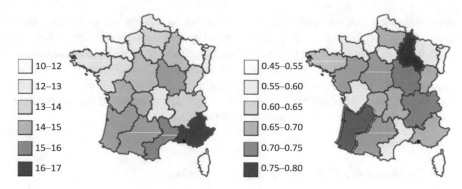

| 10–12 | | 0.45–0.55 |
| 12–13 | | 0.55–0.60 |
| 13–14 | | 0.60–0.65 |
| 14–15 | | 0.65–0.70 |
| 15–16 | | 0.70–0.75 |
| 16–17 | | 0.75–0.80 |

**Fig. 2** Observapur: regional variations in human urinary disorders

For urinary disorders related to prostate adenoma the treatment time with each molecule is much shorter than the recommended time after analysis of the results of clinical research studies. The following hypothesis can therefore be formulated: for patients treated in routine practice the clinical efficacy of these drugs as perceived by the prescribing team is not as good as that published in clinical research studies.

For patients operated on for prostate adenoma more than 30% quickly resume medication for the same condition. This leads to three hypotheses: either it is a diagnostic error and the origin of the urinary disorders was not related to a prostatic obstacle but to a bladder or neurological pathology, or these patients were badly operated on, or they were operated on too late with already-irreversible bladder disorders. Whatever the reason, this result leads to questions about the relevance of the therapeutic approach leading to the surgical indication. Its main findings can only be obtained through unbiased follow-up of cohorts of patients treated in routine practice in France.

## General Reflections

The advantages of the SNIIRAM–PMSI database.

The SNIIRAM–PMSI database enables analysis of the care pathway. The follow-up of cohorts of patients treated in current practice by analyzing the data in the database enables the study of their care pathway. This type of study is particularly effective for surgical pathologies for which the surgical procedure is very structuring in PMSI and for those for which the use of drugs clearly indicates the existence of an active pathology in SNIIRAM.

The SNIIRAM–PMSI database could be a central tool for studying the efficiency of therapeutic management and could be of use in improving the current financing system in France, which cannot continue as it is today. The financing method is "blind" in that it reimburses for all hospitalizations or all procedures performed without knowing whether or not they were relevant and justified, with the known perverse effects that this has. If we want to maintain the French health insurance model it is becoming urgent to replace this blind system with a system that takes into account the efficiency of care pathways. Moreover, this requires the implementation of tools to enable, even macroscopically, this evaluation of efficiency.

Observapur's results show that the SNIIRAM–PMSI database could be a central tool for analyzing the efficiency of care, at least for surgery, provided that appropriate treatment and analysis methods are put in place.

## The Limits of the SNIIRAM–PMSI Database

The "black hole" of new surgical procedures.

The SNIIRAM–PMSI database is therefore particularly effective at analyzing the efficiency of surgical management. However, there is a major anomaly that totally prevents us from studying the efficiency of new surgical procedures. The simple reason is that it takes several years, sometimes more than 10 years, before a specific descriptive code is available when a new surgical procedure appears in France after receiving the CE marking. Take assisted robot surgery as an example: today more than 70,000 patients have been operated on in France with this technique, and yet there is no specific descriptive code to distinguish this technique from traditional laparoscopic surgery. Had a descriptive code been created as soon as this technique was introduced, we would have at our disposal all the data from the care pathway of this cohort of 70,000 patients, some of which would have been more than 10 years old making it possible to analyze the short-, medium-, and long-term surgical complications and therapeutic results of this technique and to compare it with those of conventional laparoscopic surgery.

However, beyond this absurd loss of extremely useful information necessary to better assess the current practical efficiency of these new surgical procedures, what is even more shocking is the impossibility of organizing a means of tracing the way in which new techniques are disseminated. It is precisely because they are new that they should be subject to enhanced traceability because nobody can exclude the occurrence, one day, of a Mediator-type tragedy with a new surgical procedure.

Would it be acceptable for a new drug to be marketed and sold in thousands of copies without being identified by a specific CIP code? The answer is obviously no. So why is it accepted for surgical procedures?

A solution to remedy this situation had however already been clearly identified as early as 1987 by Christian Prieur and Professor Jean-Louis Portos in their report requested by the French Prime Minister whose objective was to identify the reasons for the obsolescence of the then Nomenclature Act of France (the NGAP) and to specify the bases for creating a new Nomenclature Act. This report stressed the need to decouple the now descriptive from the new surgical nomenclature, which must be rapid and keep pace with technical progress, from the tariff now which responds to a longer process: "The clear distinction between the functions of updating the wording and pricing seems to be a condition for the proper updating of the new nomenclature.

The updating and prioritization of the wording of the NGAP has suffered from the primacy given to financial considerations over technical and scientific issues…" It is now technically possible to create precise, non-tariffed despecification codes as soon as a new surgical technique arrives in France. To overcome the blockages and put an end to this completely anomalous and prejudicial situation for all there is a need for a legitimate authority to denounce and rise up against it. This authority could be the Academy of Medicine and Surgery.

## Interpret the Data in This Database Correctly

Interpreting the data extracted from this database to make sense of them without making mistakes is complicated. The scope of this database changes over time and the nomenclatures identifying diagnoses, drugs, and procedures evolve, as do the modalities of therapeutic management. There is a need to combine technical skills with clinical skills to avoid oversights or misinterpretations. Such a tandem arrangement is essential for good interpretation of the data.

## Lack of Clinical Data

One of the limitations of the SNIIRAM–PMSI database is that it does not contain precise clinical data describing the patient's condition and stage of pathology. Flexibility in the conditions for linking this database with clinical research databases would significantly improve knowledge about the relevance and efficiency of care. This will be one of the major challenges facing use of this new NSDS database in the coming years.

## Adapted Means

To optimize and promote the use of this database it may be necessary to set up new organizations encompassing a few principles such as encouraging the sharing of processing power to facilitate its operation in a perfectly secure way, encouraging the sharing of a metathesaurus of documented requests to harmonize extractions and reduce the risk of errors, encouraging the development of new algorithmic analysis methods that no longer start from clinical hypotheses but explore without a priori the relationships between these data, and encouraging the development of new ways of representing results that make it easy to understand the patient care journey and its variants.

## Conclusion

Our experience of Observapur illustrates that the care pathway of a cohort of patients can be followed in a relevant way by analyzing data from the NSDS, a new SNIIRAM–PMSI database.

This type of cohort follow-up is essential to EBM-based clinical research if the efficiency of therapeutic management in France is to be better understood. When it comes to surgery there is an urgent need to put an end to the gap that exists in the identification of new surgical procedures. Finally, use of this database should not only be encouraged but also facilitated by encouraging the establishment of new cooperative forms of work involving engineers, technicians, and clinicians.[1] Such analyses and operations are complex, cumbersome to carry out, and the methods used today are often not powerful enough. However, current and future developments in artificial intelligence will undoubtedly enable us to achieve this, thus providing choice in public health.

# Hospital Databases

## AP-HP Clinical Data Warehouse

**Christel Daniel and Elisa Salamanca**

## Introduction

For several years the Assistance Publique-Hôpitaux de Paris (AP-HP) has been engaged in the digitization of data to offer its professionals and patients the most efficient and innovative services. This change is based in part on the overhaul and sharing of its administrative, financial, and medical information systems (in particular, the deployment of a single Electronic Healthcare Record or EHR containing all the medical data produced during hospitalizations and consultations in the 39 AP-HP facilities). The ability to uniquely identify patients and track their hospital journey over time has enabled AP-HP to build a centralized Clinical Data Warehouse (CDW) that collects medical, administrative, and social data from more than 11 million patients.

The use of clinical data provided by health professionals for patient follow-up in hospitals offers new perspectives both for the management of hospital activity and performance and for clinical research, innovation, and health monitoring or training. Applications based on artificial intelligence (AI) algorithms are multiplying (particularly, in the field of epidemiological surveillance, medical imaging, signal analysis, etc.) and make it possible to consider the implementation of predictive and personalized medicine.

In view of the ethical and societal issues raised by the creation of the CDW and these new uses, operating rules developed in cooperation with the medical community and patient representatives make it possible to define the conditions necessary for accessing data and carrying out projects. AP-HP has also undertaken significant work

C. Daniel (✉)
Data and Digital Innovations Department—Information Systems Direction AP-HP, LIMICS INSERM UMRS 1142, Paris, France
e-mail: christel.daniel@aphp.fr

E. Salamanca
Data and Digital Innovations Department—Information Systems Direction AP-HP, Paris, France
e-mail: elisa.salamanca@aphp.fr

© Springer Nature Switzerland AG 2020
B. Nordlinger et al. (eds.), *Healthcare and Artificial Intelligence*,
https://doi.org/10.1007/978-3-030-32161-1_8

57

to ensure regulatory compliance making the CDW the first hospital warehouse for clinical data with CNIL (Commission Nationale de l'Informatique et des Libertés) authorization in France.

To enable the development of innovative research projects (particularly, in AI) AP-HP decided to set up its own IT infrastructure integrating storage and computing capacities to ensure the secure and efficient use of the huge quantities of health data for which it is responsible. Significant efforts are being made to remove a number of methodological and technological obstacles (anonymization and interoperability of data, automatic language processing tools, data quality, etc.) to enable these technologies to develop in a way that respects patient privacy.

## Issues and Uses of the Health Data Warehouse

The Clinical Data Warehouse (CDW) was set up to provide AP-HP professionals with a tool to improve the management of hospital activity and advance scientific research in the field of health by promoting multicenter data studies, supporting clinical trials, and developing decision support algorithms.

Clinical data provided by doctors, caregivers, and automatons as part of patient follow-up (medical and paramedical observations, imaging data, medical prescriptions, results of biological examinations, etc.) are sources of extremely valuable information. The possibilities offered by digital advances, such as text and data mining, statistics, machine learning, and deep learning, open up new perspectives (in particular, enabling the development of predictive and personalized tools).

## *Improve the Management of Activity and Hospital Performance*

By making it possible to cross-reference data produced in the context of care with administrative and financial data the CDW facilitates the management of hospital and medicoeconomic studies. Hospital managers and senior executives have dashboards to monitor the relevant indicators they have defined on the activity or performance of their services. For example, it is possible to monitor patients' journeys and the modalities of their care within a department, a hospital establishment, or at the more general level of AP-HP and to adjust accordingly the hospital's care offer. Services can also assess more specifically the geographical situation of their patients, the complications encountered, and waiting time before obtaining an appointment from a more organizational point of view. The long-term challenge is to enable the evaluation of hospital performance and to be able to transparently communicate the level of quality of care provided to patients. Thus, use of the CDW will make it possible to evaluate the impacts of certain strategic decisions on organizations or the quality of care (consequences of the shift to ambulatory care, creation of a new center, etc.).

Analyzing correlations between hospital data and external data, such as weather events or pollution episodes, would also make it possible to anticipate in real time peak periods in emergencies and act more quickly when triggering appropriate measures.

The implementation of activity-based pricing that, on the one hand, allows the analysis of statistical links between detailed information on the patient's journey and diagnostic codes and procedures used during coding, on the other hand, can be used to automatically detect codes or to search for missing codes. Visibility over the patient's entire stay makes it possible to better understand care pathways and define typical patient profiles.

The prospects offered by the CDW for hospital management are very important. The implementation of predictive tools thanks to the development of AI in this field opens up new opportunities that could potentially affect the way hospital organization is designed.

## *Facilitate Epidemiological Research and Data Studies*

Data research only uses data already collected, does not involve the participation of patients, and does not change the way caregivers manage them. Although data studies could have been carried out before implementation of the CDW, the various data sources had to be integrated individually in conjunction with each service concerned thus hindering the conduct of large-scale multicenter studies. By ensuring the integration of data upstream the CDW makes it possible to facilitate and develop these projects. Epidemiological studies made possible by access to hospital data are extremely varied. In particular, it is possible to carry out prevalence studies, analyze comorbidities or the causes of certain pathologies, carry out prognostic studies to analyze the future of patients who have undergone specific surgery, for example, or to evaluate professional practices. The presence of economic and financial data also makes it possible to integrate a medicoeconomic dimension into these studies.

The use of CDW data will also make it possible to carry out real-life studies the importance of which was highlighted by the Polton–Bégaud–von Lennep report.[1] Pharmacoepidemiology and pharmacovigilance of hospital data, possibly cross-referenced with data from national medicoadministrative databases (SNIIRAM, PMSI, etc.), have emerged in recent years. In particular, it is possible to monitor the safety, use, or efficacy of health products put on the market. Compliance analysis also makes it possible to consider new ways of financing drugs and medical devices.

---

[1] Bégaud B., Polton D., von Lennep F., "Les données de vie réelle, un enjeu majeur pour la qualité des soins et la régulation du système de santé," May 2017, p. 105.

## Facilitate Intervention Research

In addition to conducting data studies the CDW can also facilitate intervention research. By preceding clinical trials with a feasibility study the number of patients meeting a set of inclusion and exclusion criteria can be identified. For example, a clinical trial evaluating the efficacy of a drug needs to identify the patients for whom the drug being evaluated is indicated based on analyzing the hospital's clinical and biological data. The CDW system includes a transversal query tool that greatly facilitates feasibility studies and consequently the conduct of clinical trials. Its impact on the recruitment and inclusion of patients in clinical trials is currently being evaluated. By improving patient recruitment in the current highly competitive international environment the CDW offers an important lever enabling AP-HP patients to benefit from the latest scientific discoveries.

The conduct of clinical trials also requires the completion of electronic Clinical Research Forms (eCRFs) for each patient. Reentering clinical and biological information today requires many resources and is a source of errors. The structuring and standardization of data within the CDW makes it possible to envision automatic transfer of data from the CDW to eCRFs. Resources freed up in this way could focus on data quality and analysis. AP-HP is involved in Electronic Healthcare Record to Electronic Data Capture (EHR2EDC) systems, a European project to accelerate clinical research through the reuse of hospital data.[2]

## Development of Artificial Intelligence and Decision Support Tools

AI applications are set to grow in the health sector, identified as one of the four priority areas for the development of these technologies in France.[3] AP-HP is thus developing two main areas of work aimed at building data-processing tools on CDW and at developing the use of AI both in medical decision-making support and in hospital management.

Using statistics or AI technologies allows the data processing of heterogeneous, massive, and unstructured data to be improved for storage in the CDW. These technologies make it possible, for example, to automatically extract information from data that would otherwise be difficult to use such as unstructured data, high-frequency signals, and images. Projects are principally aimed at designing text-mining tools using natural language processing (NLP) algorithms. Such tools applied to discharge summaries provide easy access within the CDW to information useful to clinicians and researchers. Another example is to use these algorithms to anonymize hospitalization reports by automatically detecting potentially identifying data within texts.

---

[2]https://www.eithealth.eu/ehr2edc.

[3]Villani C., "To give meaning to artificial intelligence: For national and European strategies," March 2018: https://www.aiforhumanity.fr/pdfs/9782111457089_Report_Villani_accessible.pdf.

Automatic or semiautomatic extraction of information and data pseudonymization or anonymization are prerequisites to the creation and large-scale exploitation of learning datasets essential for the development of decision support algorithms. There are many avenues being explored for the development of such algorithms (particularly, in the fields of intensive care, imaging, and improvement of care processes). For example, an ongoing project is investigating the prediction of osteoporotic fracture risk using an algorithm that automatically calculates bone density from abdominal scans. Research teams are also working on machine learning algorithms (neural networks) to better detect cancers by using imaging data (mammograms, tomosyntheses) or blood test data.

AI is also an important lever for hospital management and process improvement. Algorithms making possible automated precoding of hospital stays as part of activity-based pricing could provide significant productivity gains. Implementing tools to predict traffic and waiting times in emergency rooms would allow the way such rooms are organized to be adapted to offer better patient care.

To promote the development of this type of project, AP-HP organizes large-scale events around thematic topics. The Datathon for Intensive Care (DAT-ICU) held in January 2018 in conjunction with the MIT Lab for Computational Physiology was a real success bringing together more than 150 doctors and data scientists around the CDW infrastructure and an open US database (MIMIC dataset) and gathering the identified health data of 40,000 patients admitted to intensive care units.

## Regulatory Framework and Governance Put in Place

### Regulatory Framework

Primarily intended for the general management of AP-HP professionals the CDW was authorized by the CNIL on January 19, 2017. This allowed AP-HP to physically build the IT infrastructure centralizing hospital data and to authorize a certain number of purposes of use for its professionals. A declaration of compliance with the MR004 reference methodology concerning data research was reworked. This completed the system and avoided a study-by-study approach with the CNIL for those complying with the methodology.

### Organization and Comitology

The Information Systems Directorate is in charge of operational implementation of the CDW in conjunction with the Clinical Research and Innovation Department. Operating rules were developed in close collaboration with the medical community and with the participation of patient representatives. The CDW is thus based on specific governance with operational, legal, and strategic levels involving medical staff, researchers, patient representatives, and data protection officers.

## Definition of Operating Rules

The medical community was widely consulted in 2015 to define the operating rules of the CDW concerning access to data, study execution, publications, compliance with the rules of the French Data Protection Act, patient information, and consideration of the ethical dimension. Patient representatives and qualified ethics personnel were also consulted. These rules were approved in September 2016 by the AP-HP Medical Committee, the Executive Board, and the General Management of AP-HP.

A Scientific and Ethics Committee (SEC) was set up within AP-HP mainly tasked with scientific and ethical evaluation of research projects exploiting CDW data.

Healthcare professionals within care units have open access to data concerning the patients they directly care for. On the other hand, large scale studies requiring access to patient data from patients managed by multiple care teams within the same hospital or even from different AP-HP hospitals should systematically be submitted for approval to the SEC. The investigator wishing to carry out the study then writes a scientific protocol specifying the objective of the study, the data being sought, and the methodology used. The investigator must also inform all the departments that collected the data necessary for the research. Research projects within the framework of a reference methodology that have been the subject of a global declaration of conformity do not require additional steps. On the other hand, if access to nominal data is necessary or if a link with national medical and administrative databases such as the National Health Data System (NSDS) or other cohorts is envisioned, then a request for CNIL authorization must be made. Authorization of the study by the SEC does not allow the investigator to deviate from these regulatory formalities.

Access to the CDW by partners outside AP-HP such as academic organizations, associations, and industrialists but excluding insurance and financial institutions is possible under certain conditions. They must be associated with an AP-HP principal investigator and supervise the collaboration through a contract that specifies the terms of the partnership.

To ensure the security and protection of patient data in the context of data research, data processing is carried out by authorized persons explicitly identified in the access request and exclusively on AP-HP's secure IT infrastructure, which makes it possible to accurately track data access.

## Patient Information and Ethical and Societal Dimensions

As part of regulatory compliance and to ensure patient transparency a major retrospective information campaign was conducted in 2017 comprising patients admitted to AP-HP. It involved more than 500,000 patients by email and post. Individual information is now provided (explicitly in reports, in the welcome booklet, and in posters in waiting rooms) to all patients admitted to AP-HP. Details about the CDW and its purposes are also provided along with a procedure for patients to exercise their right to object. To complete the system a transparency portal has been set up on the internet. It provides patients with a description of the studies currently being carried out in the CDW and the possibility to object online to their data being processed. Regularly updated frequently asked questions (FAQs) prepared in collaboration with AP-HP professionals and user representatives are also available on the site.

The large-scale use of hospital data for research and innovation raises questions from various stakeholders such as health professionals, patients, and citizens. Such questions are identified and debated within the AP-HP's Ethics Orientation Commission and in hospitals at the level of dedicated working groups.

## Clinical Data Warehouse Information Technology Infrastructure

To meet the governance and usage challenges already mentioned AP-HP has set up an internal Big Data platform and a software suite making secure and efficient use of the health data it holds possible (Fig. 1).

### High-Performance Infrastructure, Secure Storage, and Calculation

The administrative and health data collected during patient admission, consultation, or hospitalization are gradually being integrated into the CDW. Such data mainly come from the AP-HP EHR, but there are several hundred other clinical applications.

The challenge for AP-HP is to set up an infrastructure with significant storage and computing capacities to meet the challenge of Big Data exploitation and set the stage for the emergence of innovations capable of taking advantage of recent developments in AI.

CDW storage solutions are based on a hybrid architecture combining a relational database (PostgreSQL) and NoSQL solutions. The NoSQL has now freed us from the constraints of relational databases and offers performance adapted to Big Data analysis. However, the Structured Query Language (SQL) is far from being abandoned and tools have adapted to maintain SQL access to data for data scientists (NewSQL tools).

Ensuring the platform's computing capacity (particularly, for Big Data analysis of medical images) requires implementing a computing cluster and high-tech components such as graphics processing unit (GPU) processors. They allow parallelized

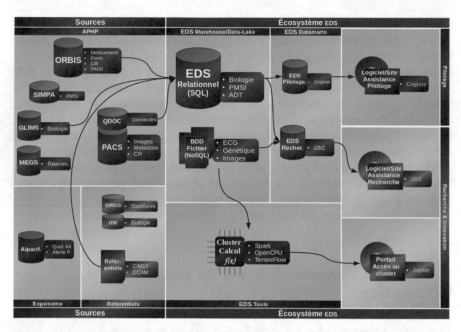

**Fig. 1** CDW system associating a high-structure infrastructure, computing capabilities, and innovative solutions dedicated to various uses such as hospital management, research, and innovation

mathematical operations to be performed accelerating data processing using automatic learning algorithms. Installed resources can be adapted (from about 10 to several hundred GPUs depending on the case) to the requirements of studies according to datasets mobilized and algorithms.

Implementation of such an infrastructure (network, servers, storage, applications, and services) represents a very costly investment in hardware, software, and human resources. People with the specific skills required for the administration of data center infrastructures are hard to come by.

The security of the CDW system is ensured at the hardware, software, and organizational levels. Indeed, an authorization matrix compliant with data access and exploitation rules, as well as solutions ensuring data confidentiality, have been put in place. In particular, data pseudonymization initially implemented on structured data has been extended to medical images and textual documents allowing their use in data research (in accordance with the MR004 reference methodology). Solutions to the complete anonymization of data and the creation of synthetic datasets are currently being found to enable innovation and use in teaching through open data.

## Solutions Dedicated to Operational Management

The Cognos solution (IBM) already used by managers centrally and at hospital centers has been updated and integrated into the CDW system. This makes it possible to offer users located closer to healthcare professionals extended functionalities to monitor activity and performance over a larger data perimeter.

## Solutions Dedicated to Research and Innovation

In a technological context marked by significant digitization with production of very high throughput data, by increased storage and computing capacities, and by the emergence of new AI technologies, an environment has been made available to researchers and digital health actors to help them use data to innovate.

It is therefore a question of setting up the technological conditions necessary to develop statistical models and algorithms to generate new knowledge from the data; evaluate the quality of the knowledge and/or models generated; develop applications that jointly exploit data and knowledge that are easily accessible by target users; and evaluate the efficiency of decision support based on AI algorithms. The open-source Informatics for Integrating Biology and the Bedside (i2b2) solution whose development is coordinated by the i2b2 tranSMART Foundation has been adopted by several hundred university hospitals worldwide.[4] Used since 2009 at the Hôpital Européen Georges-Pompidou (HEGP) and in clinical research units of AP-HP, it has also been deployed in all 12 hospital groups of AP-HP since 2016. This solution provides secure access to CDW data to identify patient populations fitting the eligibility criteria of studies (patient cohorts). The i2b2 solution associated with Jupyter, a portal dedicated to the programming of analysis solutions adapted to Big Data, makes it possible to build secure working environments for each research project. These solutions allow authorized investigators to gain easy, secure, and efficient access to the data necessary to carry out research regardless of the type of data (structured data, clinical documents, medical images, resuscitation data, monitor data, etc.).

The CDW system provides the necessary conditions for new AI technologies to emerge by facilitating data research and the development or evaluation of AI algorithms. This technical system is complemented by being able to mobilize the medical and scientific expertise needed to define research hypotheses, build learning datasets, enrich them (data annotation), and evaluate the performance of algorithms.

---

[4]Murphy S., Churchill S., Bry L., Chueh H., Weiss S., Lazarus R. et al., "Instrumenting the health care enterprise for discovery research in the genomic era," *Genome Res.*, September 2009; 19(9), 1675–1681.

## Objectives and Next Steps

Despite the progress already made many methodological, organizational, and technological obstacles need to be overcome to allow the uses planned to flourish. In particular, it is a question of developing applications capable of transforming the practices of professionals to the benefit of the health of citizens.

To make the data available as complete as possible the AP-HP aims to integrate much more such as data generated by the patient himself, data connected to the patient, environmental data (exposure data), and omics that the new bioinformatics platform centralized to AP-HP will generate and structure. The integration of such data scattered over various systems developed in non-communicating silos will require setting up a standardization chain based on the adoption of standard models and terminologies. This work undertaken in the field of data interoperability will make it possible to integrate hospital and community care data at regional and national levels to have a more complete view of the health journey of patients. The challenge is also to facilitate the integration of AP-HP into regional, national, or international research or health-monitoring networks.[5,6,7] In addition, AP-HP is committed to an approach in which data quality is evaluated and improved, which is essential to both care and research. This quality approach will be extended to the evaluation of models and algorithms generated from the data.[8]

At the regulatory level AP-HP will continuously ensure that the new services offered by the CDW comply with regulations (in particular, the European General Data Protection Regulations or GDPR).

Alongside the technical and regulatory challenges the efforts made to set up governance around data access to ensure the adoption of operating rules and the appropriation of CDW by AP-HP professionals need to be continued. One of the main challenges is to strike the right balance between the confidentiality of individual data essential to patient privacy, on the one hand, and the openness of data to advance research for the public good, on the other.

In addition to initial training in use of the tools and ongoing communication, data scientists have recently been recruited and placed within hospital groups to support health professionals and researchers to exploit data and implement new studies. Moreover, AP-HP will continue its efforts to inform patients and citizens about the opportunities provided by the CDW and about measures put in place to guarantee the confidentiality of their data and to respect their rights.

[5]Hripcsak G., Duke J.D., Shah N.H., Reich C.G., Huser V., Schuemie M.J. et al., "Observational Health Data Sciences and Informatics (OCDWI): Opportunities for Observational Researchers," *Stud Health Technol Inform.*, 2015, 216, 574–578.

[6]McMurry A.J., Murphy S.N., MacFadden D., Weber G., Simons W.W., Orechia J. et al., "SHRINE: Enabling nationally scalable multi-site disease studies," *PloS One*, 2013, 8(3), e55811.

[7]De Moor G., Sundgren M., Kalra D., Schmidt A., Dugas M., Claerhout B. et al., "Using electronic health records for clinical research: The case of the EHR4CR project," *J Biomed Inform.*, February 2015, 53, 162–173.

[8]Huser V., Kahn M.G., Brown J.S., Gouripeddi R., "Methods for examining data quality in healthcare integrated data repositories," *Pac Symp Biocomput*, 2018, 23, 628–633.

# Conclusion

As part of its digital transformation program AP-HP has committed itself to the construction of a Clinical Data Warehouse (CDW) integrating administrative and medical data from more than 8 million patients hospitalized or consulted within the 39 AP-HP facilities. The challenge facing this data warehouse, which is at the heart of the Big Data and Decision-making program of AP-HP's information system master plan, is to offer new perspectives both for the management of hospital activity and performance and for the development of research, health innovation, health monitoring, and initial and ongoing training of health professionals. The Big Data and Decision-making program has required the implementation of specific governance at operational, medical, scientific, and strategic levels involving health professionals, researchers, and patient representatives and is based on three pillars: technological, regulatory, and ethical and societal. AP-HP has decided to host within it a secure platform equipped with storage and computing capacities sized for expected use and setting the stage for the emergence of AI applications in health. The uses of CDW are gradually developing whether in the form of activity-monitoring dashboards or data research. More than 20 studies undertaken by the CDW have been authorized to date by the Scientific and Ethical Council. These are additional to the clinical trial feasibility studies or projects to develop or validate algorithms for decision support in the fields of medical imaging, resuscitation, or coding of medical activity. The main challenge facing the CDW today is to ensure that AP-HP professionals and users take ownership of the subject and imagine new uses to build the medicine of tomorrow.

# Experience of the Institut Curie

Alain Livartowski

## Introduction

As is the case in other sectors health will benefit from technologies resulting from Big Data and artificial intelligence. Cancer is one of the pathologies that will benefit most because it is a very diverse family of diseases. Since some cancers constitute just a few hundred cases in France this forces research teams to share and exchange to better treat patients and make progress in research. It is up to hospitals to ensure the preservation of data over time, measure data quality, secure data, and come up with disease modeling—all essential steps to making data interoperable and to applying AI techniques.

## Massive Amounts of Data at the Institut Curie

Cancer is a common disease generating large volumes of data in multiple formats. In addition to the frequency of procedures, consultations, and hospitalizations the management of a cancer patient requires imaging tests for diagnosis, follow-up, multiple samples, and sometimes sequencing data to study somatic or constitutional genetics.

The Institut Curie Hospital Complex made the switch to digital technology at the beginning of the 2000s, which enabled Curie Data Resources (CDR) to start printing the file in 2004 and printing radiological films in 2007. In terms of data volume this corresponds to more than 10 million medical reports, more than 100 TB of radiological images, more than 1 million images of digital pathology, and 40 TB of virtual slides to which must be added a petabyte of sequencing data. Such data

A. Livartowski (✉)
Institut Curie—Ensemble Hospitalier, Paris, France
e-mail: alain.livartowski@curie.fr

© Springer Nature Switzerland AG 2020
B. Nordlinger et al. (eds.), *Healthcare and Artificial Intelligence*,
https://doi.org/10.1007/978-3-030-32161-1_9

are variable, structured, textual, or in the form of images. Digitization in hospitals is primarily intended to improve the care process in such areas as information sharing, prescriptions, traceability, and compliance with protocols. Processes are often organized in silos that communicate little with each other and were not designed for multiaxial cross-sectional analysis for research purposes. The most enlightening example is National Information System Inter Plans Health Insurance (SNIIRAM), the purpose of which is to enable the management of health insurance beneficiaries and to study drug interactions. However, this database is unique in the world and can be used as a monitoring or pharmacovigilance tool for hospitals embarking on artificial intelligence (AI), a source of data of considerable importance.

To enhance the potential of information a new entity has been created at the Data Department of the Institut Curie. This department is responsible for setting up the necessary tools and possible cooperation to exploit the potential offered by high-volume data processing and the possibilities offered by AI techniques.

The strategy adopted by the Institut Curie is based on the following three principles: setting up an IT infrastructure enabling storage and the computing power required; making data accessible to doctors and researchers, formatting data, and linking data in warehouses to present them to AI algorithms; and cooperating with academic structures, start-ups, and manufacturers on specific projects within a well-defined scope to demonstrate that AI can provide new opportunities for research and patient care.

This revolution cannot come from hospitals alone and requires cooperation with specialists in the field. However, hospitals have a major role to play from digitization to storage, formatting, and securing data. It is also up to hospitals to inform patients so that they are aware research is being carried out on their data and that strict respect is being given to protecting the privacy of individuals. Since hospitals cannot possibly be expected to have the necessary skills in mathematics and AI techniques there needs to be cooperation with academic structures, start-ups, and industrialists.

## Data Warehouses

A data warehouse is where information is stored and conceptual links are made to enable queries, data extraction, or statistical analysis. Warehouses can be distributed or centralized, and this choice has an impact on the possibilities of data analysis and processing.

It is an illusion to think that simply copying raw data is enough to make possible an analysis of large volumes of data. For example, adjuvant chemotherapy treatment for a primary tumor or metastatic disease may be based on the same drug combination but correspond to completely different situations that would be inappropriate to group together without considering the evolutionary context of the disease.

Any conceptual data model is dependent on the database management system that supports the warehouse. It can be hierarchical, star shaped, relational, model based, or graphically oriented. Moreover, the choice depends on many criteria. Using the same

**Table 1** Data warehouses at the Institut Curie

| ConSoRe | BioMedics | ConSoRe+ | i2b2 | CDR |
|---------|-----------|----------|------|-----|
| Unicancer | Curie Institute | Curie Institute | Open source | Curie Institute |
| TLN | – | TLN | – | – |
| noSQL | RDBMS | RDF/OWL | RDBMS | RDBMS |
| Innovative | Proven | Research development | Proven | Innovative |
| User | Expert | Expert | User | User |
| Clinical research | Translational research | Clinical research | Clinical research | Fundamental research |

*CDR* Curie Data Resources; *noSQL* not only SQL; *OWL* Web Ontology Language; *RDBMS* relational database management system; *RDF* Resource Description Framework; *TLN* natural language processing

data sources the Institut Curie decided to build several warehouses to meet different objectives. The goal was to make it possible for all kinds of questions to be asked and to extract structured data for sharing between research structures or between Cancer Control Centers (CCCs). It must also be possible to take advantage of the possibilities opened up by AI to consider new analyses by means of visualization tools that will enable doctors to appropriate them.

The warehouses currently in use or under construction are ConSoRe, BioMedics, ConSoRe+, i2b2, and CDR. The characteristics of the various warehouses are summarized in Table 1 where the project promoter is indicated in line 2, the possibility or not of performing natural language processing on the warehouse in line 3, the type of database used in line 4, the innovative nature in line 5, the level of expertise of the user in line 6, and the objectives assigned to the warehouse (clinical, translational, or fundamental research) in line 7.

The ConSoRe project initiated by Unicancer aims to create a data warehouse in each Centres de Lutte contre le Cancer en français (CLCC) and to allow queries to be made in multicenters according to the principle of distributed databases. The first proof of concept showed that it was possible to launch remote requests with excellent response times, but the quality of results was too poor to meet the requirements of clinical research. It was necessary to modify the architecture of the system, replace some "bricks," design a cancer disease model capable of being adopted by all, and improve the quality of the results. It was also necessary to reconsider the human–machine interface. ConSoRe is based on the full-text elasticSearch search engine (based in Lucerne) with automatic indexing that can be classified as a noSQL search engine. This tool is therefore similar to the Google search engine that allows high-performance text searches, aggregated results in the form of facets, and search that is limited by the number of indexes. The number of indexes for CDR is limited to three: the patient, the tumor, and the sample.

The ConSoRe+ warehouse enables finer representation of the disease to better organize, better exploit the data, and above all interact with Web resources such as

Gene Ontology based on the Resources Description Framework (RDF) model. This model opens the door to the Semantic Web and offers greater query capabilities based on the SPARQL language.

The BioMedics warehouse is based on a relational database management system (RDBMS) enriched with data structured in ConSoRe and integrating biological data. It is used as a bridge between clinical and translational research. The data are structured with strongly typed attributes, and reality is modeled to fit into a model based on set theory to apply algebraic and logical operations. The tool makes possible, for example, dynamic annotation of blood or tissue samples (fixed or cryopreserved).

CDR is a data warehouse dedicated to research. This warehouse enables various research teams to organize, describe, and manipulate the data they have at their disposal. The warehouse does not itself aggregate the data but collects descriptive metadata associated with their physical location. Data collected are of various kinds such as results of molecular biology analyses (WES, WGS, RNAseq, CGH, etc.) carried out on biological samples from the hospital or from outside the hospital. Data from analyses performed on laboratory animals, isolated cells, and microscopy images are also included. Clinical annotations supplement such research data where available. CDR is a collaborative space that allows transversal vision of the data assets available to be had. The data are stored in each research laboratory or on dedicated infrastructures of the information system, but it is possible to know which examinations have been carried out and on which samples. The warehouse is a platform that subject to rights and projects enables collaboration between research teams. A direct link with consent information is provided in the case of research projects involving humans.

The i2b2/tranSMART/SHRINE suite is implemented in most US university hospitals and is gradually spreading to many academic sites including Administration of Paris Public Hospitals (AP-HP). Interest in this warehouse is growing because it is opening up the way to multicentric studies by sharing anonymized cohorts for collaborative research. The user interface is simple and intuitive, but queries can only be made on data structured in a hierarchical star model.

## Text Information

Despite wanting to structure patient records at the source more than 80% of CDR data is in text form (essentially, in medical reports). Until recently it was difficult to hope to generate any exploitable informational value from such data. Progress in this area is very rapid using techniques such as the extraction of information by so-called "cartridge rules of knowledge" or "semantic cartridge" rules. The quality of automatically structured information is highly variable, sufficient for data mining, but still insufficient for use in clinical research or care. To improve the structuring of medical reports or to extract knowledge AI techniques such as supervised learning can be used.

Taking a piece of text from a consultation report as an example a free-text medical report can be constructed as follows: "stopping letrozole according to the patient's wishes due to poor tolerance." The term "letrozole" is indexed because it is found in a drug repository; it becomes so-called inferred and structured data and is the "coding" part of the sentence. The rest of the sentence is the "non-coding" part indicating in this example that processing has been stopped. Such words act as regulatory "genes" that make the coding part inactive. It is therefore necessary in a report to take into account semantics and context as well as coding and non-coding—much like the case in genetics.

Progress in automatic language processing must be combined with image analysis, which will allow all available information to be taken into account and will represent a real step forward.

## Images

The automatic analysis of medical, radiological, nuclear medicine, or anatomopathological images is one area where the impact of AI can clearly be seen. Computers can see what the human eye does not see; moreover, they learn. Algorithms can be used to assist in diagnosis, prognosis, or prediction of responses to treatment. Although machines are not designed to compete with experienced radiologists or pathologists, some diseases are rare and difficult to diagnose and a diagnostic aid can help in getting the right questions asked. Using machines for boring and tedious tasks can save time and increase reproducibility. It is in the field of predictive or prognostic factor analysis that the contribution of AI will be major because it takes into account longitudinal monitoring of the disease.

## Example of Ongoing Projects

Currently, the work carried out at the Institut Curie on AI is still at the research level and is not yet used in clinics. Research projects in AI based on asking clinical questions are being carried out by the Data Department in cooperation with start-ups or academic structures.

The Similar Case Project in association with the start-up Owkin consists in starting with a patient's file and searching for patients having the same clinical and evolutionary profiles found in all medical texts. The goal then is to create practice based on the principle of evidence-based medicine derived from clinical studies such as randomized clinical trials. However, there are many situations where we do not have such studies, and doctors often have to rely on their clinical expertise. The principle of similar cases relies on cases stored in the memory of computers and hence becomes collective memory in contrast with individual memory.

The Cancer and Thrombosis Project consists in classifying thromboembolic disease as a previous disease, a circumstance of cancer discovery, or a complication. The second step involves identifying known risk factors. If we find known risk factors in an unsupervised learning model published in the medical literature, then it will be possible not only to identify new risk factors but more importantly to analyze the interactions between these various risk factors.

The Comedication Project aims to understand nègative or positive interactions between certain therapeutic classes and cancer drugs with the objective of ascertaining the histologically complete response rate of patients treated with chemotherapy. This type of research is only possible if we have large volumes of structured data, hence the need to partner with health insurance in the use of SNIIRAM data.

Another project in association with the start-up Sancare consists in using natural language processing techniques to help code diagnoses and procedures for the Medicalization of In-training Systems Program (PMSI) or to automatically code a tumor identity card using machine learning tools.

Many projects are underway or about to start concerning the automatic analysis of radiological or anatomopathological images such as analysis of the texture of mammary magnetic resonance imaging (MRI) to predict the response to neoadministrative chemotherapy; automatic screening for breast cancer by mammography or early screening for hepatic metastases of uveal melanoma by MRI; research on imaging genomic correlation in the neuroblastoma of children; assistance with pathological diagnosis using machine learning tools for round cell and spindle cell tumors; and research into prognostic factors using automatic analysis of virtual slides during longitudinal patient follow-up in many types of cancer.

## Conclusion

The use of Big Data and AI technologies for health still poses many challenges such as which databases should be used for supervised learning. In addition to the important question about the quality of databases it must be understood that training databases for certain diseases vary over time, that new treatments (targeted therapy, immunotherapy) are changing the history of cancer, and that the classification of cancers is constantly evolving thanks to advances in biology.

Other important questions concern how to ensure the appropriateness of the results by the doctor, how to visualize the results, what degree of confidence can be placed in the results, and what experiments and clinical studies will be needed to answer such questions.

# Knowledge by Design

Jean-Yves Robin

Any exploitation of health data requires above all exploitable data irrespective of whether they comprise decision-making information, artificial intelligence, or more traditional analyses. This apparent truism has serious implications that must be measured.

Data are real raw material on which potential prospects offered by their use depend. Moreover, having a unique national heritage of health data would be a necessary condition for France to become a leader in this field. Although such a condition is probably not enough, it would give France a considerable competitive advantage. However, data that are "poor" or difficult to access constitute an indisputable handicap or could even make any attempt at competition illusory.

It is this observation that led the French government to launch the Health Data Hub initiative in the country.

## What Is the Diagnosis for France?

There are four types of health data:

- *Medicoadministrative data*—wherein products are mainly produced by invoicing systems for inpatient and outpatient care;
- *Care production data*—produced by health professionals and the technical devices they use for care, prevention, and screening activities (such so-called real-life data are a valuable source that benefits from the expertise of health professionals);
- *Research data*—such as cohort data and registries on various pathways or on clinical trials; and

J.-Y. Robin (✉)
Impact Healthcare, Paris, France
e-mail: jy.robin@impact-healthcare.fr

© Springer Nature Switzerland AG 2020
B. Nordlinger et al. (eds.), *Healthcare and Artificial Intelligence*,
https://doi.org/10.1007/978-3-030-32161-1_10

- *Patient data*—produced by patients themselves under various circumstances including without their knowledge.

These different areas must be examined in terms of their quality, on the one hand, and their availability, on the other. Medicoadministrative data have the merit of being centralized and by and large cover the entire French population. It is a considerable achievement for France to have had centralized data on the whole population since 1999. Although still underutilized, such data are already being used to monitor drug consumption or detect disease outbreaks. Recent establishment of the Health Data Hub aims to develop the use of such data. Nevertheless, there is still room for improvement in view of the many possible fields of application of data sciences in health. They are mainly used for the invoicing of procedures—not the search for new therapies or the evaluation of care. France's competitive edge remains modest on this point. It is not widely known that France has the largest health database in the world in the National Information System Inter Plans Health Insurance (SNIIRAM). Although this is correct in terms of claim collection, it is clear that US advances in precision medicine and innovative therapies involve more than just the analysis of insurance claims. The rapid collection of data from electronic healthcare records (HERs) will allow new capacities within the next few years. Data on the delivery of care depend on a long process initiated some 20 years ago as a result of the computerization of health professionals through the equipment of private practitioners and the computerization of hospitals. This process is now hampered by well-known challenges. For hospitals there is the real complexity and heterogeneity of business processes, governance issues, the weakness of the resources available or devoted to computerization, and the management of change that should accompany it. For the private practitioners the challenges include assimilating computerization to administrative tasks and value-creating processes and an economic model that is not conducive to the development of coordination of care and other tasks that could support such computerization resulting in poorly or not documented patient files managed using often inefficient software resulting from an underfunded sector.

Research data are either held by public research organizations and therefore generally not very accessible except to academic research teams, or private data on the work of pharmaceutical companies. The lack of public–private cooperation programs in France and the historical compartmentalization of clinical and research data are challenges facing the development of translational medicine.

Finally, there are data produced by patients themselves. Such data are often captured by major US digital players or have emerged through early uses of connected devices. It should be noted that the French language represents only a small percentage of messages sent internationally, but natural language processing solutions are now very efficient.

## Public Policies Favoring Data

Strong public support is a prerequisite to developing the health data analysis sector and its promising applications. Such public support in favor of the production of data in exploitable forms and the facilitation of data access by both public and private actors can be carried out through such actions as:

- Enrichment of billing flow data to open up opportunities to evaluate care and change business models used for professional remuneration.
- Structuring data according to semantic repositories based on what has been successfully achieved with medical synthesis and Pluridisciplinary Consultation Meeting forms as part of the shared medical file in 2013.
- Deployment of the National Health Record (DMP) and the possibility of using its data for research and evaluation of care—not just for coordination.
- Clarifying the status of data produced during care (access to which cannot be decided upon request but must be facilitated and regulated in a transparent manner).
- Major efforts in terms of interoperability by promoting semantic repositories on the main medical disciplines (to which the colleges of specialties could contribute).
- Value creation in the production of data by health professionals should be taken into account in exchange for the obligation to make such data available in the public interest. Data whose production is mainly financed by the public national health insurance must be used without misuse in the general interest. However, the time spent by these same professionals to document their actions must be included in remuneration since producing relevant data is an integral part of the delivery of care.
- Use of the new General Data Protection Regulation (DGPS) to simplify procedures for accessing data and strengthen the rights of individuals thus fully reflecting the spirit of the DGPS; and
- Deployment of a global patient information policy giving people the real opportunity to object to the use of their personal data according to the main purposes of the use of such data (care delivery, clinical research, medico-economic evaluation...) and respect for everyone's wishes.

A significant source of value creation would be to take into account at the design stage of health information systems their technical, legal, and economic capacity to produce usable data and sources of new knowledge. Such a "knowledge by design plan" could provide the fertile ground we need to support innovation based on health data.

# Diagnosis and Treatment Assistance

# Artificial Intelligence to Help the Practitioner Choose the Right Treatment: Watson for Oncology

**Christine Garcia and Georges Uzbelger**

## New Era of Information Technology

We have entered a third era of computing: the era of artificial intelligence. The first was made up of non-programmable machines that performed very simple calculations on digital data. Users of these machines interpreted the results obtained to generate information. The second comprised today's massively used computers allowing the processing of information via computer programs developed according to business needs. Users employ the results to generate knowledge from their experience and the associated context. The third was initiated by IBM in 2011 and is related to the phenomenal amount of data and information humans produce and use. Since these can be structured or unstructured (currently nearly 80%), only a machine equipped with artificial intelligence can produce knowledge effectively for users in their business.

The bioinspired approach entails machines with artificial intelligence learning and being inspired by our methods of reasoning.

These machines are artificial intelligence agents developed to achieve business objectives based on data and information collected and generated. Depending on the case some artificial intelligence techniques require the use of machine or deep learning algorithms that can be broken down into initial training and learning steps (supervised, unsupervised, reinforced, or competitive learning).

C. Garcia (✉) · G. Uzbelger
Syntec Numérique Santé, Paris, France
e-mail: christine.duval@fr.ibm.com

G. Uzbelger
e-mail: georges.uzbelger@fr.ibm.com

© Springer Nature Switzerland AG 2020                                          81
B. Nordlinger et al. (eds.), *Healthcare and Artificial Intelligence*,
https://doi.org/10.1007/978-3-030-32161-1_11

## From Descriptive and Predictive to Prescriptive

These artificial intelligence systems enable decision-makers to make more objective decisions based on descriptive analyses (e.g., symptoms) and predictive analyses in an inductive generalization process (e.g., diagnosis and prognosis). These decisions are the result of prescriptive analyses (e.g., medical prescriptions) such that actions appropriate to the expected results taking into account business rules can be carried out.

These systems are thus valuable decision-making tools for humans who as a result become more objective.

## IBM Watson Solution

IBM Watson is a perfect example of systems with artificial intelligence.

IBM Watson for Oncology was initially designed in 2013 with the help of the Memorial Sloan Kettering Cancer Center to assist in the diagnosis of breast and lung cancers and is being expanded in 2018 to 13 types of cancers including bladder, liver, prostate, and esophagus.[1]

This solution is currently deployed in 155 facilities in 12 countries around the world to assist healthcare professionals to identify the most appropriate therapeutic protocol for 45,000 patients.

It is based on evidence extracted and interpreted from the patient's clinical record, treatments now available and reflected in national recommendations, clinical studies, specialized scientific publications, and sources for adapting recommendations to possible drug interactions.

More than 15 million pages and 300 medical journals (published primarily by ASCO, EBSCO, Elsevier, MMS, NCCN, Wiley, and PubMed) are analyzed by Watson for Oncology. It does so by implementing data and text-mining algorithms that perform digital and non-digital data processing (structured and unstructured) and natural language understanding. Carrying out this analysis on an ongoing basis the system provides the relevant information and knowledge necessary for health professionals to carry out their activities and enables them to free up considerable time.

Watson for Oncology is a decision-making tool for the practitioner and is used before and during multidisciplinary consultation meetings (MCP) to determine the best treatment by the physician. Watson for Oncology has a 93% agreement rate with healthcare professionals on treatment choice for breast cancer (ref).

---

[1] https://www.ibm.com/watson/health/oncology-and-genomics/oncology/ and https://www.mskcc.org/about/innovative-collaborations/watson-oncology.

## Prospects for the Future

Systems equipped with artificial intelligence, machine learning techniques, and high computing power make possible the statistical processing of large amounts of structured and unstructured data and thus open up new health applications that were previously unimaginable.

Possible applications include diagnostic assistance, diagnostic tools, recommendations for treatments such as Watson for Oncology, physical medicine, and rehabilitation assistance. As clinical data become increasingly accessible in unprecedented volumes statistical analyses on such large cohorts of patients can now be combined to identify subpopulations that respond in different ways, identify comorbidities, measure the effectiveness of various protocols, etc.

We are seeing the arrival of platforms that now make it possible to search for anomalies in medical imaging data (thus facilitating screening and improving diagnosis), to process genetic data (Watson for Genomics[2]), and to carry out epidemiological studies and client-based trials (Watson for Trial Clinical Matching[3]).

In addition to assisting the physician in making treatment choices direct patient assistance is a real application of these techniques. For the treatment of chronic diseases it is the patient who is in continuous charge of his or her treatment and who makes daily decisions that can impact her or his condition.

In general, new data will be able to assist healthcare workers in caring for patients with disease. From such previously unavailable data new decision-making tools using artificial intelligence techniques will emerge to help citizens, patients, families, caregivers, and medical staff to prevent problems as far as possible before they occur and even to propose solutions to counteract bad evolutions in patients' health status.

For example, to allow fragile people who do not have a close family to live independently in their homes surveillance technologies to observe their activity in a nonintrusive manner can be put in place for security purposes. The addition of learning systems means these same technologies can assist in prevention and prescribing.

---

[2]https://www.ibm.com/watson/health/oncology-and-genomics/genomics/.

[3]https://www.ibm.com/watson/health/oncology-and-genomics/oncology/.

# Artificial Intelligence to Help Choose Treatment and Diagnosis Commentary

Jacques Rouessé and Alain Livartowski

Some industrial firms have quite legitimately embarked on using the capabilities of artificial intelligence (AI) to bring indisputable elements to the diagnosis and treatment of cancer. Such legitimacy is based on correlations that can be established by the use of Big Data and on the observation that practitioners cannot control all the data that regularly appears in the field of their specialty or on the precision that digital image processing can provide. For example, machines can facilitate the selection of relevant publications from the literature sparing practitioners from time-consuming bibliographic and graphic research that they are far too busy to complete.

Although the help of such a system at the semiology level may seem to be little more than an accessory, it is not the same for digital imagery data the analysis of which can go as far as the interpretation of cytological or histological data. It is also this technology that will make possible reading the constitutional or somatic genome essential for targeted and personalized therapy. Thanks to information from the literature, decision trees, automatic image analysis, and genome data, machines should be able to suggest prognostics-related diagnoses or therapeutic attitudes that can, for example, guide prescription-adjuvant therapy to prevent the emergence of metastases.

The development of such a system can only be conceived within the framework of close collaboration between computer scientists, biocomputers, specialists in charge of diagnostic and therapeutic management, clinicians, radiologists, pathologists, biologists, and geneticists. Collaboration between IT manufacturers, cancer control institutions, and university hospitals is essential.

However precise and sophisticated the algorithms may be, this device should only be considered as an aid to the care of a patient whose responsibility can only be assumed by a doctor. The latter must bear in mind that the algorithms involved,

J. Rouessé
Académie nationale de Médecine, Paris, France

A. Livartowski (✉)
Institut Curie, Paris, France
e-mail: alain.livartowski@curie.fr

© Springer Nature Switzerland AG 2020
B. Nordlinger et al. (eds.), *Healthcare and Artificial Intelligence*,
https://doi.org/10.1007/978-3-030-32161-1_12

whether or not their learning is supervised, will necessarily have limited relevance because their development is artificial. For example, literature analysis does not necessarily imply that published data are more valuable because they are published in a journal with a high impact factor. In addition, positive studies are published while studies that do not show superiority over a reference treatment are not published. The number of publications is certainly considerable and hence there is a lot of data available that it is important to identify, classify, and use; it is here that machines can be of great help. However, this does not apply to a patient who has exhausted all the therapies evaluated in the literature, who has a progressive disease, who requires a new effective treatment, and for whom there are no clinical studies to guide the practitioner. Here it is not the case that there is too much data but insufficient data. This is where the analysis of "real-life" data can be interesting but needs to be applied with the prudence and critical thinking that is more characteristic of humans than machines.

Clinical data may vary and be incorrectly recorded; for example, if the physician notes a particular clinical sign that suggests a diagnosis, it is because he or she often has the diagnosis in mind. Imaging also has its limitations because its interpretation must always take into account the context. It should be kept in mind that even histology does not always have an absolute value and must be compared with other data contributing to the diagnosis. As for the prognosis, it is at best only a "truth" that will never be anything but statistical.

Assessment of the performance of such a system depends on the cancer and takes into account tumor locations, histology, stage, and genetic data. For example, breast cancer management is well codified by easily accessible recommendations and the decision on the initial treatment regimen generally requires little discussion. It is understood that concordance here between the opinion of such a system and that of specialists may be greater than 90%. However, in the remaining 10% of cases there are elements such as the social context, the patient's psychology, and the assessment of possible comorbidities and toxic risks that are sources of difficulties and discussions. If treatments are well codified at the beginning of cancer disease, then the more advanced the disease (since multiple therapeutic lines are available) the fewer the evidence-based medical recommendations and the fewer the identical cases based on experience.

Another fundamental point is that therapeutic attitudes are closely linked to the health system. Thus, management can be different from one hospital to another without being able to say which one achieves the best results. Management of a patient in the United States, France, and India is different because the available means cannot be compared. The algorithms must take this into account; they cannot be exported without taking into account the context because medicine is not universal.

The use of AI in oncology has to face up to the diversity of life, the randomness of evolution, environmental factors, host characteristics, chaos theory, the pressure exerted by therapeutics in evolution of the disease, and changes induced by such therapeutic advances. Thus, predicting the future based on past data is difficult enough, but it would be paradoxical if it were a brake on innovation.

The diversity of life is like an abyss and the deeper we progress in our knowledge of the genome, the biology of systems, the interactions between the host and its environment, and the ability of life to adapt the more we understand why a doctor never meets two patients with exactly identical symptoms. Our knowledge of biology and theories on the physiology of life and physiopathology have evolved at a prodigious rate in recent years. Thus, our knowledge and certainties have only a very relative value, and the history of medicine shows us how much we must remain modest in the face of disease, even though our treatments are ever more effective. So, predictions based on past events should encourage us to be very humble, a quality that we should learn from computers and that a good doctor should maintain.

Finally, there is the concern that absolute faith in such machines may lead non-specialists to believe that they are competent to manage pathologies with which they are only seldomly confronted and for which they will not have sufficient critical thinking skills based on experience. Studies will therefore have to be carried out to provide scientific proof of the usefulness of such machines in daily practice. It is also necessary to consider the difference between implementing a new technique, using and adopting it in practice, and seeing it spread.

The golden rule for the use of AI in medicine and oncology, in particular, is that it must take into account that part of human beings that is immeasurable. The best example is that if the notion of connected patients is already proving fruitful for both patients and caregivers, it is because these connections are only effective if there is a close dialogue between caregivers and other caregivers who have previously established the personalized "rules of the game" for monitoring.

We would like to share the enthusiasm and optimism of the coauthors of the previous chapter who predict a new era. The chapter suggests that problems can be solved when we are at the beginning of a patient history—a probable revolution in medicine but one full of pitfalls and technological, scientific, and ethical obstacles. As is often the case with new technologies their implementation in practice will face difficulties. Experience should help to overcome them. The reservations we have expressed simply indicate that we will have to evaluate the help we will receive from such systems. All the fruit that can be expected from them will probably ripen later than expected, and it is likely that they will generate surprises that are positive rather than negative.

# Medical Imaging in the Age of Artificial Intelligence

Nicholas Ayache

Artificial intelligence is disrupting the world of medical imaging. Algorithms and models that are already very present in the construction of medical images are now powerful enough to guide the analysis of medical images as well as—if not better than—human experts. These algorithms allow the construction of digital representations of the patient that guide diagnosis, prognosis, and therapeutic management. On May 2, 2018 a symposium at the Collège de France brought together many experts on this subject. Their contributions are visible on the Collège de France website.[1,2]

In dermatology a deep convolutional network previously trained on more than 1 million natural images was then adjusted with the images of 130,000 dermatological lesions. It could automatically distinguish cancerous lesions from benign ones as well as an expert dermatologist. In radiology the French company Therapixel developed a deep convolutional network of 640,000 mammograms in response to a global challenge and won the competition by distinguishing suspicious mammograms from normal ones better than all its competitors. Its software now surpasses the performance of expert radiologists. Finally, in ophthalmology other deep convolutional networks trained on more than 130,000 images of the retina are able to detect diabetic retinopathy as well as an expert ophthalmologist. For the first time in history software (IDx-DR) has been approved by the Food and Drug Administration (FDA) to make this diagnosis automatically without the image being seen by an ophthalmologist.

Even though these results are spectacular, they remain for the moment confined to specific, relatively narrow tasks on which there are huge databases previously

---

[1] Berry G., "Medical imaging and machine learning: Towards an artificial intelligence?": https://www.college-de-france.fr/site/gerard-berry/symposium-2017-2018.htm.

[2] Ayache N., "Digital Patient and Artificial Intelligence," Collège de France, May 2, 2018: https://www.college-de-france.fr/site/gerard-berry/symposium-2018-05-02-02-09h05.htm.

N. Ayache (✉)
INRIA, Sophia Antipolis, France
e-mail: nicholas.ayache@inria.fr

© Springer Nature Switzerland AG 2020
B. Nordlinger et al. (eds.), *Healthcare and Artificial Intelligence*,
https://doi.org/10.1007/978-3-030-32161-1_13

labeled by experts. However, these databases are not numerous and their acquisition (especially, their labeling by experts) is very expensive. It is necessary to ensure that rare cases (which by definition are not numerous!) are well represented, that there is no bias (gender, age, ethnicity, etc.), and that there are enough healthy subjects (which poses an ethical problem when the imaging modality is irradiation, for example). Collecting such databases and making them available to learning algorithms also raises serious confidentiality issues.

Moreover, artificial intelligence is not limited to the development of deep convolutional networks whose millions of parameters are difficult to interpret and whose adjustment requires training on huge databases. There are a variety of classification algorithms that can be trained on databases of very variable sizes with very good results.[3] It is also possible to build numerical models of the patient that exploit all the knowledge available in anatomy and physiology to limit the number of more easily interpretable biophysical parameters. Finally, the computational framework of the digital patient makes it possible to synthesize medical images that are realistic enough to train automatic learning systems and then to transfer the learning to real images. Modern data science methods also make it possible to take into account increasingly "holistic" data on the patient including imaging data (structural and functional), biological data (genetic, metabolic, etc.), and even behavioral and environmental data (lifestyle, etc.). Thus, the UK Biobank database plans to make all such data acquired on more than 100,000 participants available to the scientific community.[4] In France a major project to collect image data associated with other biomedical data acquired on a very large number of patients is being implemented at Administration of Paris Public Hospitals (AP-HP) to serve the scientific community.[5]

The field of application of artificial intelligence in medical imaging is intended to serve all medical disciplines such as radiology, dermatology, ophthalmology, neurology, psychiatry, cardiology, senology, hepatology, endoscopy, endomicroscopy, anatomopathology, radiotherapy, and image-guided surgery.[6] New legal issues are

---

[3]Thirion B., "Introduction to Big Data Approaches to Medical Imaging," Collège de France, May 2, 2018: https://www.college-de-france.fr/site/gerard-berry/symposium-2018-05-02-02-09h35.htm.

[4]Nichols T., "Challenges and Opportunities in Population Neuroimaging," Collège de France, May 2, 2018: https://www.college-de-france.fr/site/gerard-berry/symposium-2018-05-02-02-11h30.htm.

[5]Beauffret R., "The databank project of AP-HP," Collège de France, May 2, 2018: https://www.college-de-france.fr/site/gerard-berry/symposium-2018-05-02-11h00.htm.

[6]Bertrand A., Durrleman S., Epelbaum S., "Neuroimaging, neurology and digital models for Alzheimer's disease," Collège de France, May 2, 2018: https://www.college-de-france.fr/site/gerard-berry/symposium-2018-05-02-14h30.htm; Thomassin-Naggara I., Clatz O., "Innovative technologies at the bedside of breast cancer screening: What future for women?", Collège de France, May 2, 2018: https://www.college-de-france.fr/site/gerard-berry/symposium-2018-05-02-02-15h15.htm; Fournier L., "Radiomics applied to cancerology," Collège de France, May 2, 2018: https://www.college-de-france.fr/site/gerard-berry/symposium-2018-05-02-16h30__1.htm; Brady M., "Some examples of transfers from laboratory to practice," Collège de France, May 2, 2018: https://www.college-de-france.fr/site/gerard-berry/symposium-2018-05-02-17h301.htm.

being raised by the emergence of new decision support software[7] and questions are being raised about the very future of certain medical specialties.[8] All these applications and issues are addressed in many other chapters of this book.

To conclude I would like to stress that artificial intelligence and the digital patient should be regarded as computer tools at the service of 4P medicine based on the four fundamental principles of personalization, prediction, prevention, and participation so that patients can receive better treatment. These new tools are intended to help doctors—not to replace them. Indeed, some of the physician's qualities such as compassion, comprehension, critical thinking, and professional consciousness (the 4Cs) are still and will for a long time be the prerogative of human intelligence. They remain irreplaceable today.

---

[7] Trick D., Potier de la Varde B., "The lawyer's questions: What protections for patients and data?", Collège de France, May 2, 2018: https://www.college-de-france.fr/site/gerard-berry/symposium-2018-05-02-12h00.htm.

[8] Besse F., "Why do radiologists have hopes and fears with AI," Collège de France, May 2, 2018: https://www.college-de-france.fr/site/gerard-berry/symposium-2018-05-02-18h00.htm.

# Artificial Intelligence in Medical Imaging

Johan Brag

## Artificial Intelligence in Medical Imaging: Drivers

### *Precision Medicine*

We are witnessing a paradigm shift in healthcare from a standard treatment model to a model that takes into account individual variability of response to treatment (namely, precision medicine). The objective of precision medicine is to provide the best available care to each individual based on stratification of patients according to their phenotypes or biological profiles. Such personalized medical care designed to benefit patients requires the acquisition of clinical information from various sources such as imaging, pathology, laboratory tests, and genomic and proteomic data to optimize treatment. In general, such clinical information is extracted and measured from quantitative biomarkers that act as substitutes for the presence or severity of a disease such as blood pressure, heart rate, and other measurements.

As a result of its widespread clinical presence medical imaging is ideally positioned to play a central role in medicine including screening, early diagnosis, assessment of treatment response, and probability of recurrence of various cancers.[1]

---

[1]Giardino A., Gupta S., Sepulveda K. et al., "Role of imaging in the era of precision medicine," *Acta Radiol*, 2017, 24, 639–649.

---

J. Brag (✉)
Median Technologies, Valbonne, France
e-mail: johan.brag@mediantechnologies.com

© Springer Nature Switzerland AG 2020
B. Nordlinger et al. (eds.), *Healthcare and Artificial Intelligence*,
https://doi.org/10.1007/978-3-030-32161-1_14

93

## Medical Images as a Source of Clinical Data

Information from medical imaging systems such as scanners comprises more than just sources of images for visual interpretation by a radiologist; they also provide a rich source of clinical data that are often difficult for a human observer to process.[2] In medical imaging a large number of biomarkers have been defined, often empirically, to measure the progression of a pathology such as cancer. Initially measured manually, they are now frequently extracted and assessed automatically or semiautomatically using increasingly sophisticated image-processing software.[3]

Thousands of parameters can be extracted from medical images by analyzing morphological, functional, and textural characteristics that can then be statistically correlated with the genotypes and phenotypes of various tissues.[4] This information can then be merged with radiological signatures and interpreted by experts for diagnostic or prognostic purposes[5] using methods similar to face or fingerprint comparison methods.

In the near future it is likely that many medical images will be generated specifically for analysis assisted by artificial intelligence (AI) systems rather than visual interpretation by a physician. Some imaging techniques such as ultrasound elastography or magnetic resonance imaging (MRI) spectroscopy already produce numerical data rather than images.

# First-Generation Artificial Intelligence Systems

Although not specifically referred to as AI tools, medical imaging computer-aided diagnostic systems have been in existence for more than 20 years. These systems often lacked the computing power now available in the cloud and the algorithms were shallower (in terms of complexity) than current learning algorithms, but the overall architecture was often the same.[6]

---

[2]Gillies R.J., Kinahan P.E., Hricak H., "Radiomics: Images are more than pictures, they are data," *Radiology*, 2016, 278(2), 563–577.

[3]Parmar C., Leijenaar T.H., Grossman P. et al., "Radiomic feature clusters and prognostic signatures specific for lung and head and neck cancer," *Sci. Rep.*, 2015, 5, 11044.

[4]Lambin P., Rios-Velazquez E., Leijenaar R. et al., "Radiomics: Extracting more information from medical images using advanced feature analysis," *Eur J Cancer*, 2012; 48(4), 441–446.

[5]Aerts H.J.W.L., Velazquez E.R., Leijenaar R.T.H. et al., "Decoding tumor phenotype by noninvasive imaging using a quantitative radiomics approach," *Nat Commun*, 2014.

[6]Lee G., Lee H.Y., Park H. et al., "Radiomics and its emerging role in lung cancer research, imaging biomarkers and clinical management: State of the art," *Eur J. Radiol*, 2017, 86, 297–307.

## Automatic Analysis of Medical Images

The first medical image analysis systems appeared around 1990 and were generally based on mathematical models that were highly dependent on human knowledge. The methods focused mainly on organ segmentation, image registration over time and between modalities, lesion detection, and size[7] measurement.

The models were often not generalizable and were of low predictive value. Diagnosis was generally made visually and mostly based on the appearance of lesions with various morphological properties or using empirical models to differentiate between benign and malignant lesions. Phenotypic features (image characteristics) were generally described visually and the radiologist interpreted the results to arrive at a diagnosis. For example, in lung cancer screening the descriptors of visual appearances evolved over time and the categories only roughly corresponded to specific risk profiles. Ambiguities in terminology, a lack of standardization of methods, and significant variability in interpretation between observers limited the accuracy of these systems. The characteristics extracted from the images also tended to be non-specific in terms of malignancy significantly increasing the number of false positives.[8]

## Quantitative Medical Imaging

Since the early 2000s medical imaging has gradually become more quantitative because of the capability of extracting objective and measurable characteristics for the statistical assessment of the severity, degree of change, or status of a disease compared with a previous study or normal pathology. Quantitative imaging includes the discovery, development, and optimization of imaging biomarkers; standardization of acquisition protocols; data analysis; and results display and reporting. These advances have made it possible not only to set up a reference clinical database but also systematic monitoring of certain pathologies such as lung cancer.[9]

Such databases will eventually make it possible for patients to be treated according to their individual characteristics.

---

[7]Doi K., "Computer-Aided Diagnosis in Medical Imaging: Historical Review: Current Status and Future Potential," *Comput Med Imaging Graph.*, 2007, 31(4–5), 198–211.

[8]Coroller T.P., Grossman P., Hou Y. et al., "CT based radiomic signature predicts distant metastasis in lung adenocarcinoma," *Radiother. Oncol.*, 2015, 114(3), 345–350.

[9]Ginneken B., Schaeffer-Prokop C.M., Prokop M. et al., "Computer-aided diagnosis: How to move from the laboratory to the clinic," *Radiology*, 2011, 261(3), 719–732.

## *Radiomics*

The sequencing of the genome at the beginning of the century profoundly changed all diagnostic methods (especially, in the field of medical imaging). One of the major drivers in the growth of medical imaging is projected to be systematic large-scale analysis of data from imaging examinations. Radiomics is a recent discipline in that it emerged around 2010. It is based on systematic mining of clinical, biological, molecular, and genetic data contained in medical images.[10]

Radiomics is the process of extracting multidimensional data from medical images acquired from computed tomography (CT), magnetic resonance imaging (MRI),[11] and positron emission tomography (PET) using image-processing algorithms. Recent studies have shown that quantitative data derived from medical images such as shape, size, tumor volume, signal strength, attenuation, and texture can be used as biomarkers to predict treatment response.[12] In radiomics medical images containing information on tissue pathophysiology are transformed into digital data that can be used at the large scale for diagnosis and prognosis. Such data can then be processed using Big Data and AI[13] analysis systems.

Radiomics approaches have been validated for diagnosis and prognosis, prediction of treatment response, and disease surveillance and monitoring (particularly, in oncology).[14] Radiomics has helped to further the original objective of precision medicine: the creation of prevention and treatment strategies that consider individual variability through the analysis of large datasets such as medical images, demographic and clinical data on patients, pathology, biological tests, and genomic sequences. The success of precision medicine is largely dependent on the discovery and development of robust quantitative biomarkers. Medical imaging, non-invasive and accessible in routine clinical practice, is an important source of such biomarkers.[15]

---

[10]Lee J., Narang S., Martinez J. et al., "Spatial habitat features derived from multiparametric magnetic resonance imaging data are associated with molecular subtype and 12 months survival status in glioblastoma multiforme," *PLoS One*, 2015, 10(9), e0136557.

[11]Gevaert O., Xu J., Hoang C.D. et al., "Non-Small Cell Lung Cancer: Identifying prognostic imaging biomarkers by leveraging public gene expression microarray data—Methods and preliminary results," *Radiology*, 2012, 264(2), 387–396.

[12]Lambin P., Leijenaar R.T.H., Deist T.M. et al., "Radiomics: The bridge between medical imaging and personalized medicine," *Nature Reviews Clinical Oncology*, 2017, 14, 749–762.

[13]Lao J., Chen Y., Li Z.C. et al., "A deep-learning-based radiomics model for prediction of survival in glioblastoma multiforme," *Sci. Rep.*, 7, 10353.

[14]Limkin E.J., Sun R., Derclerk L. et al., "Promises and Challenges for the implementation of computational medical imaging (radiomics) in oncology," *Ann of Oncol*, 2017, 28, 1191–1206.

[15]Van Ginneken B., "Fifty years of computer analysis in chest imaging: Rule-based, machine learning, deep learning," *Radiol Phys Technol*, 2017, 10, 23–32.

## Searching for Information Within Images

Analyzing correlations between pathophysiological information and images requires the creation of automatic methods for large-scale extraction and indexing of image characteristics in search engines. Traditionally, only metadata associated with images were accessible through a search of image databases. Following the development of radiomics it is the information contained directly in the pixels of the images that has to be analyzed and compared. New types of search engines capable of directly querying image content—content-based image retrieval (CBIR)—such as Median Technologies' iBiopsy have been developed precisely for this task (Figs. 1 and 2).

A first-signature extraction engine segments the liver that is then automatically divided into "tiles" corresponding to a tissue sample (virtual biopsy). For each tile a large number of features such as texture are extracted from the images. A measure of similarity makes it possible to visualize these features and correlate them with biological factors such as the malignancy of certain tumors.

These characteristics are then indexed as signatures in databases stored in the cloud (Fig. 3).

A second search engine makes possible direct comparison between signatures corresponding to a given patient with a reference database of tens of thousands of

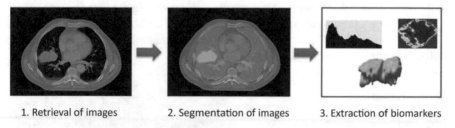

1. Retrieval of images     2. Segmentation of images     3. Extraction of biomarkers

**Fig. 1** Illustration of the radiomic process

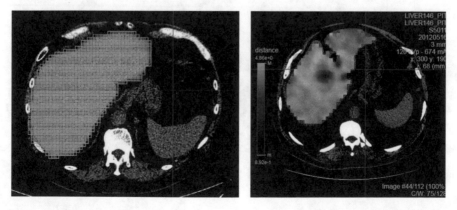

**Fig. 2** Extraction of textual characteristics from images

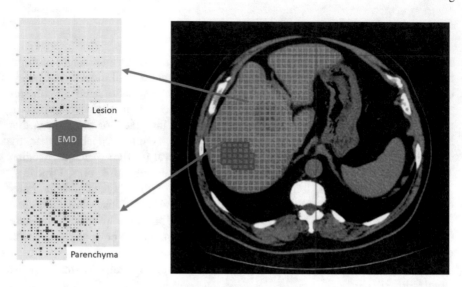

**Fig. 3** Automatic extraction of radiological signatures

patients with a similar pathology. The results can then be filtered according to criteria such as age, genetic or biological test results, and other clinical data (Fig. 4).

A third data analysis engine produces an analytical dashboard that predicts membership in a specific phenotype class or predicts disease progression based on statistical analyses of patients with similar profiles.

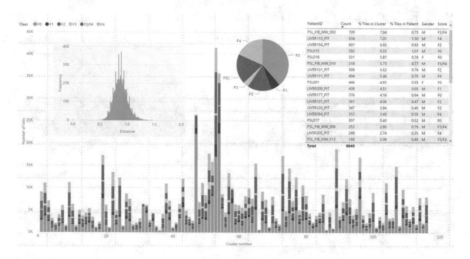

**Fig. 4** Analytical dashboard

## Deep-Learning Revolution

In parallel with the development of systems for assisted driving and object detection in photographic images, deep-learning image- processing methods appeared around 2012. The novelty of these methods rests in their independence of the vocabulary used to define the characteristics of images. Rather than being limited to a predefined number of features the system itself generates the optimal features for data classification. Having at its disposal an almost infinite number of variables such a system can theoretically model a certain pathology while taking into account variability within each phenotype, which can be massive. One of the controversial aspects of this type of model is that the specific reasoning used by the system to classify a particular image is often unidentifiable. This black-box concept has the potential to generate technical problems to correct classification errors and medical liability problems in the event of a serious diagnostic error. If it becomes impossible to assess how the system makes a decision is it the machine or the doctor who makes the diagnosis?

Despite some initial reluctance deep-learning methods have been able to achieve comparable or even better performance than experts for a large number of laborious image-processing tasks such as organ segmentation and lesion detection and classification.[16] The accelerated pace of development of new deep-learning algorithms (particularly, convolutional neural networks) combined with the increased computing power associated with cloud computing and augmented reality architectures have enabled a greater advance in medical imaging AI in the last 5 years than in the previous 30.[17] The increasing availability of open-source software and the creation of image databases for training deep- learning systems have made it possible to multiply the number of groups working on the various problems. International competitions on a given theme often bring together several thousand competitors. Countries such as China and India, until recently absent among the leaders in the field of AI, have made rapid progress and teams from these countries are regularly among the winners of these competitions.

## Supervised Learning

The first major advances in integrating AI in medical imaging were based on the use of supervised learning techniques. Such systems rely on the availability of a large number of labeled samples to train the system. The performance of these systems for relatively simple classification tasks often exceeds that of experienced radiologists. Figure 5 illustrates how these supervised learning methods can be used effectively to segment an anatomical structure. A supervised learning model is used to train an

---

[16]Litjens G. et al., "A Survey on Deep Learning in Medical Image Analysis," *Medical Image Analysis*, vol. 42, December 2017, 60–88.

[17]Aerts H.J.W.W.L., "Data science in radiology: A path forward," *Clin Can Res*, February 2018, 24(3).

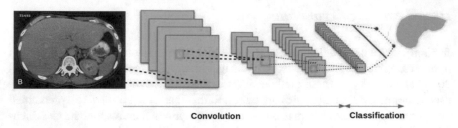

Convolution                                        Classification

**Fig. 5** Neural network used for automatic liver segmentation

algorithm to classify voxels in an image of the liver as belonging to tissues inside or outside the liver. The accuracy of the classification obtained is around 94% with a calculation time of 100 s per image.

## *Limits of Learning Systems: Curse of Dimensionality*

Despite the rapid breakthrough of AI it has not solved some fundamental problems related to the use of machine learning methods. The "curse of dimensionality" is the first of these problems.[18] Discovered by mathematician Richard Bellman in 1961 the curse of dimensionality refers to the general rule that for any system of learning a natural state from samples representative of that state characterized by a large number of variables (dimensions), the number of samples required to ensure the robustness of the system increases rapidly with the number of variables. By its very nature the quality of a deep-learning system is closely linked to the complexity of the model (i.e., the number of dimensions). A very large number of samples (medical images) is therefore necessary to predict the contribution of a feature extracted from the images to a particular pathology. Due to a shortage of samples the number of images required to achieve acceptable predictive performance is often insufficient relative to the number of features resulting in an overfitting problem called Hughes phenomenon.[19]

Hughes phenomenon limits the scalability of learning systems and requires new approaches. This problem can be partially offset by dimensionality reduction techniques the effects of which are often unpredictable.[20] Although regularization methods derived from optimal transport[21] techniques open up a number of promising avenues, they require very high computational power (Fig. 6).

The second problem relates to the fact that these systems require a large number of manually labeled images to train the system. It is often difficult in medical imaging,

[18]Bellman R.E., *Adaptive Control Processes: A Guided Tour*, Princeton University Press, 1961.

[19]Hughes G., "On the Mean Accuracy of Statistical Pattern Recognizers," *IEEE Transaction*, vol. 14, issue 1, 1968.

[20]Goodfellow I., Bengio Z., Courville C., *Regularization for Deep Learning*, MIT Press, 2016.

[21]Villani C., *Optimal Transport: Old and New*, Springer, 2008.

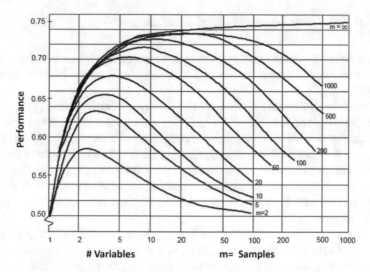

**Fig. 6** For a given number of variables the performance of a learning system increases with the number of *m* samples (see footnote 19)

sometimes even impossible, to obtain previously labeled images when the ground truth is unknown.[22]

## A Potential Alternative: Transfer Learning

Training a learning system from scratch is difficult because it requires a large number of labeled images for training and a significant amount of expertise in the field to ensure that the model converges properly. A promising alternative is to refine a learning system that has already been developed on images taken from another field of medical imaging or acquired from another modality.[23] However, substantial differences between medical images of different modalities can make such a knowledge transfer difficult. The transfer of knowledge from one type of scanner image to another is more likely to be successful than the transfer of knowledge from MRI images to scanner images, for example. Nevertheless, this approach does not solve the fundamental problem of the limited number of prior-labeled images.

[22]Thrall J.H., Li X., Quanzheng L. et al., *Artificial Intelligence and Machine Learning in Radiology: Opportunities, Challenges, Pitfalls and Criteria for Success*, American College of Radiology, 2017.
[23]Tajbakhsh N., "Convolutional Neural Networks for Medical Image Analysis: Full Training or Fine Tuning?", *IEEE Transactions on Medical Imaging*, 2016, vol. 35, issue 5, 1299–1312.

## *Optimal Solution: Unsupervised Learning*

The ideal for deep-learning systems would be to use unsupervised learning methods. These are systems in which the model learns the classification itself without prior labeling.

The restricted Boltzmann machine (RBM) is a type of unsupervised deep-learning network. This type of learning model has been used for a number of tasks including the automatic detection of microcalcifications in digital mammography.[24] It automatically learns the features that distinguish microcalcifications from normal tissues and their morphological variations. Within the system low-level image structures typical of microcalcifications are automatically captured without any selection of features by an expert or manual preprocessing that were often necessary with supervised learning methods.

Another class of unsupervised learning networks is comprised of generative adversarial networks (GANs). Yann LeCun, one of the pioneers of deep-learning networks, recently described such types of networks as representing the greatest progress made in machine learning in the last 10 years. The method dates back to 2015, is based on game theory, and has the purpose of jointly training two antagonistic networks. One of the networks seeks to generate synthetic data as reliably as possible so that such data resemble training data. The other network seeks to distinguish synthetic images from real images as accurately as possible. The first network will therefore try to deceive the second network; hence they are in opposition or antagonistic.

A GAN can thus produce synthetic models of phenotype images that can be used to drive an unsupervised learning system. Such models have been applied to the synthesis of medical images, as well as to segmentation, detection, registration, and classification.[25] Pathological abnormalities can also be identified by unsupervised learning on large-scale imaging databases.[26] GANs can also be used to significantly increase the number of image samples to drive a learning system by, for example, generating synthetic images of lesions as shown in Fig. 7.

Interestingly, GANs generally outperform other advanced deep-learning networks for small and medium datasets, the typical situation in medical imaging.

---

[24] Seung Yeon Shin, Soochan Lee, Il Dong Yun, "Classification based micro-calcification detection using discriminative restricted Boltzmann machine in digitized mammograms," *Proc. SPIE 9035, Medical Imaging*, 2014.

[25] Frid-Adar M., "Synthetic data augmentation using GAN for improved liver lesion classification," 2017: https://scirate.com/arxiv/1801.02385

[26] Schlegl T., "Unsupervised Anomaly Detection with Generative Adversarial Networks to Guide Marker Discovery," *Proceedings of International Conference on Information Processing in Medical Imaging (IPMI, 2017)*.

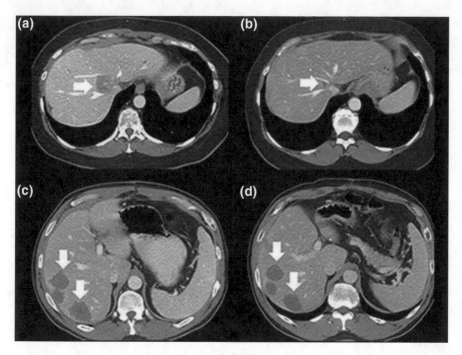

**Fig. 7** Synthetic image generation for unsupervised training. (*left*) Real lesions and (*right*) synthetic images that can be used to train the system

## Future of Artificial Intelligence in Medical Imaging

Traditionally, the interpretation of medical images has been based on human expertise alone. The increased volume of data and the greater complexity and diversity of medical images initially led to the development of computer-assisted diagnostic methods. Then, advances in radiomics made it possible to extract medical images of features correlated with the pathophysiological state of the disease and the response to treatment. Despite the wide range of known anatomical or texture-based features many diseases do not have sufficiently validated image biomarkers, while for other diseases existing biomarkers lack predictability. The deep-learning systems introduced over the past five years have succeeded in taking an important step forward enabling the system itself to generate the most predictive features. They have the potential to radically transform the delivery of healthcare, but it takes a lot of data to train them and achieve good performance. Lack of access to data is the main obstacle to their development. The first generation of supervised learning systems required a large collection of previously annotated data that limited their usefulness in medical imaging. More recent unsupervised learning techniques based on antagonistic networks offer hope for better expansion of AI to clinical routines.

# The AI Guardian for Surgery

**Daniela Rus and Ozanan R. Meireles**

## Motivation

Imagine an Intelligent Operating Room that becomes an extension of the surgeon, extending all the senses using embedded sensors, and guarding all aspects of surgery to ensure the best outcomes. The Intelligent Operating Room monitors carefully every image and action in the operating room, and is able to detect problems and issue warning to the surgeon before the problems are visible to the naked eye. State of the art computer vision systems can detect critical problems such as the potential rupture of a blood vessel with enough advance notice that preventative measures could take place, identifying the current phase of the surgery and ensuring that the right tools and people are in the room, altogether supporting decision making. The Intelligent Operating Room becomes a Guardian for the Surgeon, providing just in time actionable information and suggestions for corrective and preventative actions. In the future, the Guardian Operating Room will empower the surgeon to provide the best care to the patient, preventing mistakes and providing suggestions for acting in the most effective and optimal way. Using recent advances in developing Guardian Autonomy systems (Schwarting et al. 2018) that have introduced new algorithms rooted in data, machine learning, computer vision, and robotic technologies to implement Guardian systems for autonomous driving, we can leverage the basic algorithms and extend them to develop shared human-machine control to surgery, with machines supporting surgeons with perceptual, cognitive, and physical tasks.

D. Rus (✉)
Computer Science and Artificial Intelligence Laboratory (CSAIL), Department of Electrical Engineering and Computer Science (EECS), Massachusetts Institute of Technology, Cambridge, USA
e-mail: rus@csail.mit.edu

O. R. Meireles
Surgical Artificial Intelligence and Innovation Laboratory, Massachusetts General Hospital, Boston, USA

© Springer Nature Switzerland AG 2020
B. Nordlinger et al. (eds.), *Healthcare and Artificial Intelligence*,
https://doi.org/10.1007/978-3-030-32161-1_15

Imagine that in the future, the Intelligent Operating Room will also provide the surgeon with a range of intelligent tools for conducting procedures. Ingestible robotic mini-surgeons (Miyashita et al. 2016) will be used for a range of surgical procedures that will be performed without incisions, without pain, and without the risk of infection. Using recent advances in origami robots, a future with incision-free surgery for some procedures will be realized by creating robotic pills that can be swallowed, programmed to perform a procedure, and then dissolved when the procedure is complete. For example, an origami mini-robot can be used as a "mini-surgeon" robot to remove button batteries or other foreign objects that have been swallowed accidentally. The mini-surgeon robot will be packaged in an ice pill that gets swallowed; when it arrives in the stomach the ice melts and the robot deploys. The robot can then be controlled using an external magnetic field similar to an MRI machine to get to the battery, pick it up using an embedded magnet, and eliminate it through the digestive system. This idea if intelligent ingestible robotic tools has a wide range of applications, including obtaining tissue samples, stopping bleeding, delivering medicine to precise locations, and event get a better view inside the bodies, all of these without incisions.

On an individual patient level, the Intelligent Operating Room with its AI Guardian function will offer opportunities to make surgery safer, smaller, and more precise. That means advanced warning and intelligent tools that prevent life-threatening situations. It means intelligent support for managing challenging post-operation situations and disabilities (Katzschmann et al. 2018). It means customized healthcare, built using knowledge gleaned from enormous amounts of data. And counter to common knowledge, it means more patient-centric focus, not less, as the precision gains from AI and robotics will increase the efficiency of procedures and allow the surgeons to spend more time with their patients in post-operative situations.

On a global hospital scale, the Intelligent Operating Room and its AI Surgery Guardian function will help us generate better insights into addressing important challenges: understanding how to obtain the best surgical outcomes by collecting and analyzing data from vast wireless sensor networks that monitor the surgeon, the patient, and the tools in the operating room; improving hospital operations by data-driven decision making, scheduling, and planning; eliminating mistakes by monitoring, and training young doctors to perform like the best surgeons. It will help improve education for all doctors through monitoring and guiding procedures that are adaptive to progress, to ensure that every young doctor gets access to the skills needed to serve the patients in the most skilled way.

## Fourth Surgical Revolution

Technology has great potential to transform surgery, enabling the fourth revolution in the field. Surgery is one of the most important and broadest fields in Medicine and it is routinely performed in large numbers worldwide. The American College of Surgeons adopted the following definition for surgery: "Surgery is performed for the purpose of structurally altering the human body by incision or destruction of tissues and is part of the practice of medicine. Surgery also is the diagnostic or therapeutic treatment of conditions or disease processes by any instruments causing localized alteration or transportation of live human tissue, which include lasers, ultrasound, ionizing radiation, scalpels, probes, and needles. The tissue can be cut, burned, vaporized, frozen, sutured, probed, or manipulated by closed reduction for major dislocations and fractures, or otherwise altered by any mechanical, thermal, light-based, electromagnetic, or chemical means."[1]

The oldest reports of surgical procedures are dated from 6,500 B.C.E. where archaeological findings in France reviewed human skulls with drilled holes (a procedure called trepanation (Geddes 2003))[2]. However modern surgery only started to be developed during the late 1800s, and even though inhumane procedural pain, deadly infections, and speed over precision were common and outcomes were poor.

The history of surgery however progressed very quickly transforming medicine in general, due to key transformations introduced by disruptive "technologies". First the advent of General Anesthesia, allowed surgeons to perform all different kinds of operations in absence of pain, which resulted in a much larger application of surgical procedures, and precision start gaining predilection over speediness.

The second biggest transformation in the field of surgery was the introduction of the concept of asepsis and utilization of surgical antiseptic techniques, which markedly decreased morbidity and mortality caused by infection.

The third disruptor of the surgical practice, was the introduction of minimally invasive surgery, which markedly decreased pain, infection, and other complications associated with bigger incisions, leading to faster recovery, shorter hospital stay, and overall better outcomes. Minimally invasive surgery fundamentally relies on video processors, HD monitors, fiber optic cables, cameras, super low caliber Instruments going through trocars measuring in average 2–12 mm, use of hypersonic scalpels, advanced bipolar energy sources, staplers, suturing devices. And more recently there has been fast introduction of Master-Slave robotic actuators (Gawande 2012).[3]

We are now on the verge of the fourth revolution, with the introduction of artificial intelligence into the operating theater, with the goal of augmenting the surgeon's cognitive capabilities through the use of computer vision, natural language processing, and machine learning applications. This could greatly mitigate inherited human errors such as, eventual inadequate intraoperative decision making or inability to recognize potential anatomical variations, therefore predicting and avoiding errors before they occur. Furthermore, the connectivity of the pre-operative, intra-operative and post-operative phases of care through advanced medical records platforms will

---

[1] https://www.facs.org/~/media/files/advocacy/state/definition%20of%20surgery%20legislative%20toolkit.ashx.

[2] Geddes JF. Trepanation: History, Discovery, Theory. *J R Soc Med.* 2003 Aug; 96(8):420. PubMed Central PMCID: PMC539585.

[3] Gawande A., Two hundred years of surgery. N Engl J Med. 2012 May 3; 366(18):1716–23. https://doi.org/10.1056/NEJMra1202392.

become more fluid, and individual patient data, could be cross validated with population of data based on prior experiences, allowing surgeons to provide better predictions in the more precise recommendations of treatments back to the individual level; achieving precision medicine (Hashimoto et al. 2018a).

Goals: "This book chapter is an introduction to the field of Artificial Intelligence in Surgery, focusing in the operating room environment. This overview defines the opportunities and challenges of the use of AI in this field; discusses current applications and potential future developments, provides an overview of common technical approaches, and fundamental ideas of artificial intelligence.

Historically, surgery has always been a very conservative field, where innovation struggles to be noticed and lingers to be adopted in large scale, until it has been scrutinized by countless regulatory bodies. Usually new devices and techniques take several years before being introduced into the surgical armamentarium, and many more years before becoming widely used, and only a few of them ever thrive to become a standard of care. As discussed above, surgeons benefited from the creation of anesthesia, the development of antibiotics, and the introduction of minimal Invasive techniques, making it possible to perform a multitude of procedures ranging from simple and routine to extremely challenging and sometimes controversial ones, which were never thought to be possible decades ago.

The highly advanced minimal invasive tools, video equipment and robotization, now allows surgeons to reach spaces with extremely precision, dexterity, efficiency, and in the safest possible fashion. This set of high-tech equipment also generate a large amount of data that has been scantily utilized intra-operatively and historically discarded after the procedures. However, this extremely rich data has the potential to generate a shift in paradigm when combined with Artificial Intelligence, and provide enormous amount of precious information to physicians, pre, intra, and posoperatively, leading to cognitive enhancement, and to progressive introduction of different levels of automation.[4]

Recent advancements in Artificial Intelligence, and the synergic utilization of machine learning techniques, Computer Vision and Deep Neural Networks (DNNs) has been revolutionizing our society at many levels from social media and cognitive computing to the inception of autonomous vehicles.

A similar and perhaps more profound revolution can occur in the operative theater and beyond, generating unprecedented changes to the way medical care is delivered.

---

[4]Surgical Video in the Age of Big Data. Hashimoto DA, Rosman G, Rus D, Meireles OR. Ann Surg. 2018 Dec; 268(6):e47–e48. https://doi.org/10.1097/SLA.0000000000002493. No abstract available.

# Case Study: Predicting the Surgical Phase to Support Real Time Decision for Surgeries

Intraoperative adverse events such as accidental bowel or blood vessel laceration are estimated to occur in a fraction of operations and may be related to several causes, such as unexpected operative complexity or even operative errors. In surgical patients, up to two thirds of errors occur in the intraoperative phase of care, and 86% of errors are secondary to cognitive factors such as failures in judgment, memory, or vigilance that lead to poor decisions. In many common cases, particularly in minimally invasive surgery, these failures in judgment or vigilance can be traced back to errors in human visual perception (Ramly et al. 2015).

Artificial intelligence (AI) has been used in the past to describe or segment mostly-linear sequences of events in surgery video analysis or focus on specific decision statistical analysis without considering the operation as a whole. However, intraoperative decisions do not always follow a linear process, especially in emergency surgery or during unexpected events in elective surgery, and the context of an entire operation is often necessary to understand specific events. Current AI approaches have not fully accounted for nonlinear, conditional decision making or have emphasized analysis of specific decision junctions without accounting for overall procedural context. Surgical decision-theoretic model (SDTM) that utilizes decision-theoretic tools in AI to quantify qualitative knowledge of surgical decision making to allow for accurate, real-time, automated decision analysis and prediction. Such a model approximates the surgical phases as a hidden Markov decision process (hMDP), estimated along with patient state variables, allowing accurate and human-interpretable analysis and prediction of the surgery's progression and outcomes. It allows for incorporation of other frameworks, such as deep learning, and integration of tools to potentially boost efficiency (e.g. coresets) to maximize its potential.

We conducted a study to create an efficient automatic real-time phase recognition and video segmentation system for laparoscopic, endoscopic and robot-assisted surgery; and to propose a cost-effective blueprint for piloting the system in a real operating room environment, with minimal risk factors.

The technical approach consists of the following steps:

1. Ground truth data. We built a corpus of recorded video footage and text annotations of laparoscopic procedures performed by expert surgeons. In this study we focus on the laparoscopic vertical sleeve gastrectomy (LSG) procedure, which can be performed both manually or as a robot-assisted operation. For this study we used 10 videos of the laparoscopic vertical sleeve gastrectomy (LSG) procedure performed by expert surgeons at the Massachusetts General Hospital. The surgeons identified 7 basic phases for this procedure to be: (1) port, (2) biopsy, liver retraction, (3) omentum removal, dissection, hiatus inspection, (4) stapling, (5) bagging, (6) irrigation, (7) final examination, withdrawal (Fig. 1). For this study we assumed that the phases always occur in the specified order. Note that not all videos contain all the phases, which presents an additional challenge to

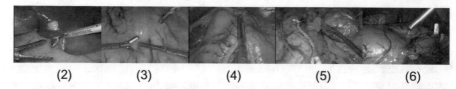

(2)            (3)            (4)            (5)            (6)

**Fig. 1** Phases of the laparoscopic sleeve gastrectomy. Phases (2–6 shown) of the laparoscopic sleeve gastrectomy (LSG) procedure: (1) port, (2) biopsy, liver retraction, (3) omentum removal, dissection, hiatus inspection, (4) stapling, (5) bagging, (6) irrigation, (7) final inspection, withdrawal

segment videos with missing phases. We then interviewed the surgeons who performed the procedures, and collected two kinds of information: (1) qualitative annotations describing how they identified the phase from the video; (2) specific timestamps of phase transitions that serve as our ground truth segmentation.

2. Frame representation. We used the ground truth data to compose a feature space that captures the axes of variability and main discriminant factors that inform the surgical phases. We used the bag-of-words (BOW) model to represent each frame. From the video annotations we identified several visual cues, categorized broadly as local and global descriptors, that inform surgeons of the current phase. We used these cues to compose a feature space of local and global descriptors that captures the principal axes of variability and other discriminant factors that determine the phase. These visual cues include color, position, shape, texture, and temporal regularity. We combine the augmented local and global descriptors into a single fixed- dimension frame descriptor. For this we use the bag-of-words (BOW) model, which is a simplifying representation commonly used to standardize the dimensionality of features (Sivic and Zisserman 2009).

3. Phase prediction. We trained a Support Vector Machine (SVM) for each phase of the procedure, introduce an observation function and Hidden Markov Model (HMM) to model the transitions and associated likelihoods, and use the Viterbi algorithm to compute the final phase prediction. As a first step, we train a series of support vector machines (SVM) for each phase. This is an iterative step that involves interviewing surgeons, re-calibrating the feature space, re-training the classifiers, and repeating the process. The second step is to make use of the temporal structure of surgical phases (monotonically increasing) to correct SVM predictions, resolve the ambiguous cases stated above, and compute a single time-series of phase predictions. Finally, we run the Viterbi algorithm (Forney 1973) on the emission sequence to find the most likely sequence of hidden states (the phases).

4. Coreset segmentation. As in our previous work (Rosman et al. 2014; Volkov et al. 2015), we computed a coreset representation of the video instead of using the entire video. Using coresets gives the same level of accuracy, while providing a computationally tractable approach that enables our system to work in real-time, and using only a fraction of the computational resources. Coresets are compact data reduction constructs that can efficiently produce a problem dependent compression of the data. As in our previous works, we use an online k-segment

coreset algorithm to compute an approximate segmentation of the video stream (Rosman et al. 2014), and construct a keyframe compression of the video based on this segmentation (Volkov et al. 2015). Using coresets allows our system to run online, in real-time, using minimal computational resources.

5. Experiments. Finally, we assessed our process with cross-validation experiments, and evaluate the performance of our system against ground truth. We assessed our system with cross-validation experiments, using both the entire video and the coreset representation, and evaluate accuracy against ground truth segmentation. We performed cross-validation tests by training the system on each subset of N − 1 = 9 videos in the dataset, using a standard 80/20 training/validation split. The system was then tested on each remaining unseen video, and the results aggregated over the N subsets. The observation function parameters were determined empirically (typical values are $\alpha = 0.8$, $\beta = 15$). The HMM transition and emission matrices learned from the data, similar to (Lalys et al. 2012). The Viterbi algorithm was run on the emission sequence to compute the final phase prediction given the outputs of the observation function. We demonstrate a 90.4% SVM prediction accuracy, and improve to 92.8% when combined with HMM. These results are on par with similar work in the surgical video domain (Lalys et al. 2010), while achieving a 90 + % coreset compression over the original video stream.

6. Potential Applications: This model also allows to obtain a statistical representation of log probability of the prediction of the next phase likelihood and can differentiate a normal and straightforward case from an abnormal one. The cumulative log probability for each frame allows real-time estimation of deviation from an expected operative path and resulted in a "surgical fingerprint" that visually summarized potential areas of unexpected operative events (Fig. 2)[5]. This model could be used for several applications, such as real time attending notification system, to notify attendings if trainees are nearing critical portion of the case or require additional assistance to complete the case; or to recommend the need of Telementoring, to establish automated communication link to human mentor when error is predicted, that could be used in battlefield as a support to medical staff who may not have specialty-specific knowledge, or rural and underserved areas in the world.

Furthermore, the uniqueness of each surgical fingerprint, as a visual representation of the output of an operation, could have some great post hoc applications such as peer review, credentialing and recredentialing, resident education, and to augment the Morbidity and Mortality conference with situation-specific video review.

We are currently extending our system to consider continuous likelihood models, allowing us use temporal regularity to handle ambivalent phase predictions more effectively. By using the learned SVMs to model log-likelihoods of the individual phases, we can obtain improved results compared to the per-frame votes while

---

[5]https://innovationblog.partners.org/getting-great-science-to-market/first-look-surgical-fingerprints-real-time-analysis-of-intraoperative-events.

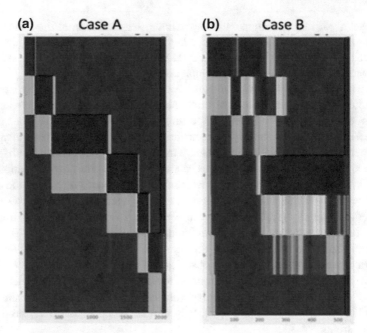

**Fig. 2** Surgical fingerprints. Comparing **a** routine sleeve gastrectomy versus **b** sleeve + lysis of adhesions

enforcing a meaningful set of transitions. To this end, we are also looking into other temporal models for non-monotonic phase sequences.

Insofar as coresets will remain a part of this project, our goal going forward would be to extend the apply the semantic video summarization framework in (Volkov et al. 2015) to create interactive visual summaries of laparoscopic and robot-assisted surgeries.

# Conclusions

The case study on predicting the next surgical phase highlights the opportunities around using machine learning and data for more effective and efficient surgical procedures. These techniques have a variety of applications including surgery state estimation from online video, partial implementation of effectors, state prediction from video, resource prediction from video, and training from video. Each of these new capabilities will take us closer to the vision of an Intelligent Surgical room providing Guardian AI support during surgery.

Machines can learn exponentially more, and by several orders of magnitude, when compare with each individual surgeon, and therefore rapidly generating a collective wealth of knowledge that will benefit each individual surgeon by augmentation of the human cognitive capabilities. This dissemination and democratization of knowledge leveraged by harnessing the unique power of Artificial intelligence and big data could lead to creation of a "collective surgical consciousness" which carries the entirety of the field's knowledge, leading to technology-augmented real-time clinical decision support, such as intraoperative, GPS-like guidance. This will undoubtedly result in improved patient care and surgeons operative experience (Hashimoto et al. 2018b).

Surgeons are well positioned to help integrate AI into modern practice. Surgeons should partner with data scientists to capture data across phases of care and to provide clinical context. Surgeons should also partner with machine learning and AI researchers for using the most advanced decision making support systems in their operations. Finally, by adding partnerships with robotics and computer vision experts, many aspects of the vision outlines in this paper to develop Intelligent Surgical Rooms and intelligent tools such as the ingestible mini-surgeons will bring the vision of Guardian AI for surgeons to serve their patience with safer and easier procedures closer to reality.

AI has the potential to revolutionize the way surgery is taught and practiced with the promise of a future optimized for the highest quality patient care.

# References

Forney GD Jr (1973) The viterbi algorithm. Proc IEEE 61(3):268–278

Gawande A (2012) Two hundred years of surgery. N Engl J Med 366(18):1716–1723. https://doi.org/10.1056/nejmra1202392

Geddes JF (2003) Trepanation: history, discovery, theory. J R Soc Med 96(8):420. PubMed Central PMCID: PMC539585

Hashimoto DA, Rosman G, Rus D, Meireles OR (2018) Artificial intelligence in surgery: promises and perils. Ann Surg 268(1):70–76

Hashimoto DA, Rosman G, Rus D, Meireles OR (2018) Surgical video in the age of big data. Ann Surg 268(6):e47–e48. https://doi.org/10.1097/sla.0000000000002493

Katzschmann R, Araki B, Rus D (2018) Safe local navigation for visually impaired users with a time-of-flight and haptic feedback device. IEEE Trans Neural Syst Rehab Eng 36(3):583–593

Lalys F, Riffaud L, Morandi X, Jannin P (2010) Surgical phases detection from microscope videos by combining SVM and HMM. Medical computer vision: recognition techniques and applications in medical imaging. Springer, pp 54–62

Lalys F, Riffaud L, Bouget D, Jannin P (2012) A framework for the recognition of high-level surgical tasks from video images for cataract surgeries. IEEE Trans Biomed Eng 59(4):966–976

Miyashita S, Guitron S, Yoshida K, Shuguang L, Damian DD, Rus D (2016) Ingestible, controllable, and degradable origami robot for patching stomach wounds. In: Proceedings of the IEEE international conference on robotics and automation, pp 909–916. IEEE Press

Ramly EP, Larentzakis A, Bohnen JD, Mavros M, Chang Y, Lee J, Yeh DD, Demoya M, King DR, Fagenholz PJ, Velmahos GC, Kaafarani HM (2015) The financial impact of intraoperative adverse events in abdominal surgery. Surgery 158(5):1382–1388. https://doi.org/10.1016/j.surg.2015.04.023. Epub 27 May 2015

Rosman G, Volkov M, Feldman D, Fisher III JW, Rus D (2014) Coresets for k-segmentation of streaming data. In: Proceedings of NIPS, pp 559–567. Curran Associates, Inc

Schwarting W, Alonso-Mora J, Paull L, Karama S, Rus D (2018) Safe non-linear trajectory generation with a dynamic vehicle mode. IEEE Trans Intell Transp Syst 19(9):2994–3008

Sivic J, Zisserman A (2009) Efficient visual search of videos cast as text retrieval. IEEE Trans Pattern Anal Mach Intell 31(4):591–606

Volkov M, Rosman G, Feldman D, Fisher III JW, Rus D (2015) Coresets for visual summarization with applications to loop closure. In: Proceedings of ICRA, Seattle, Washington, USA, May 2015. IEEE

# Toward an Operating Room Control Tower?

Nicolas Padoy

**Abstract** The modern operating room is full of data. In an age of data science and artificial intelligence, we believe that this vast amount of surgical data should be exploited to construct an AI-based surgical control tower that can model and analyze surgical processes as well as support surgical decision and action.

The modern operating room is full of data. This data is generated by various medical equipment intraoperative imaging systems, surgical instruments, and hospital information systems. More data is also generated by devices used for communication, documentation, and education such as cameras and microphones. Some of this data is already frequently processed using algorithms. For example, intraoperative images are registered to preoperative images to facilitate the guidance of the surgical procedure. Similarly, physiological data are also monitored using algorithms to trigger an alarm in the event of an anomaly. However, most of this data, such as the videos captured by laparoscopic or ceiling-mounted room cameras or the signals stemming from specific surgical equipment like electric scalpels, is currently rarely used by algorithms. This is despite the ability of such multi-modal data, taken as a whole, to describe digitally the overall progress of an operation and thus to allow the automated analysis of surgical activities.

In an age of data science and artificial intelligence, the question arises of how to use these vast amounts of surgical data to model and analyze surgical processes and to develop systems to support surgical decisions and action.[1] Like a control tower used in aeronautics the objective here is to develop a "control tower" for the operating room, as illustrated in Fig. 1.

The role of such a control tower would among other things be to facilitate real-time communication and monitoring of the progress and performance of surgical

---

[1] Maier-Hein L. et al., "Surgical Data Science: Enabling Next-Generation Surgery," *Nature Biomedical Engineering*, 2017, vol. 1, 691–696.

---

N. Padoy (✉)
ICube, University of Strasbourg, CNRS, IHU Strasbourg, Strasbourg, France
e-mail: npadoy@unistra.fr

© Springer Nature Switzerland AG 2020
B. Nordlinger et al. (eds.), *Healthcare and Artificial Intelligence*,
https://doi.org/10.1007/978-3-030-32161-1_16

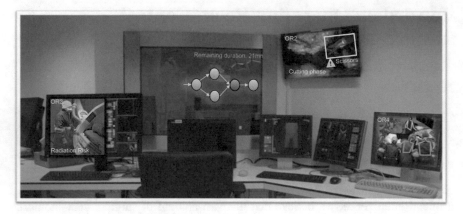

**Fig. 1** A "control tower" for operating rooms showing information on the current state of the various rooms such as the current surgical step and the risk of overexposure to radiation in hybrid surgery

procedures for all personnel concerned. This could be achieved for instance via the automated recognition of various surgical actions and other peripheral activities, the triggering of suitable reminders and alerts, and the detection of possible anomalies by comparing the data from the current procedure with data from thousands of similar procedures performed in the past. The control tower would also facilitate the development of new interfaces for human–machine interactions thanks to context recognition, for instance by selecting and transmitting relevant information to the appropriate person at the time when it is required.

Ultimately, such a surgical control tower would have the potential to facilitate the organization of operating rooms, reduce the risk of disruptions or errors, and help manage the huge amounts of data available, thus providing a new intelligent assistance tool. It would also enable the development of new tools based on objective data analysis for the comparison of good practices, process optimization, and education.

This chapter looks at two possible applications for operating room control towers. The applications were developed in the ICube Laboratory at the University of Strasbourg in collaboration with the Nouvel Hôpital Civil, the Institute of Image-guided Surgery (IHU Strasbourg), and the Research Institute against Digestive Cancer (IRCAD). Both are related to intraoperative medical imaging. The first uses information from cameras installed in the room and from an X-ray imaging system to visualize and analyze in real time the risk of overexposure to radiation. The second consists of using videos from laparoscopic surgery to automatically recognize the activities performed, index the data, and generate predictions.

## Monitoring Irradiation Risk in Hybrid Surgery

Since the number of procedures using X-rays are constantly growing, operating room room staff are increasingly exposed to radiation. Despite the protective measures in place such as the use of lead shielding and exposure control using chest dosimeters, several studies have shown that there is a risk of overexposure to certain areas of the body.[2] This risk depends, in particular, on the type of procedure, the parts of the body considered, and the positioning of personnel and equipment. Because of the large number of parameters influencing the propagation of radiation, it is difficult for an exposed person to obtain an accurate picture of the risk of exposure and the dose received at various locations in the room and in the body. To compensate for this lack of information we propose an augmented reality-based system to visualize the radiation in 3D.[3] Thanks to a set of cameras installed on the ceiling of the operating room and information provided by a robotic C-arm the positions of the equipment and personnel can be determined. This then makes it possible to simulate the 3D propagation of radiation from the emission source and, in particular, to estimate backscattering from patients that directly affects clinicians positioned around them. The resulting 3D exposure map can then be viewed in augmented reality from the camera images, as shown in Fig. 2.

Integrating such a system in operating rooms would not only make it possible to detect the intraoperative risks of overexposure to radiation, but also to train staff about these risks in an intuitive way. In addition, many extensions are possible. For

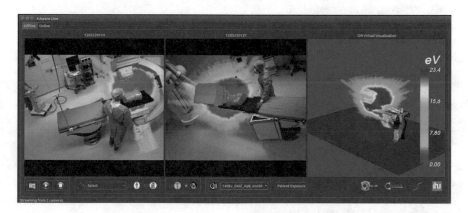

**Fig. 2** Prototype showing radiation exposure in a hybrid room using augmented reality

[2]Carinou E., Brodecki M., Domienik J., Donadille L., Koukorava C., Krim., Nikodemova D., Ruiz-Lopez N., Sans-Merce M., Struelens L., Vanhavere F., "Recommendations to reduce extremity and eye lens doses in interventional radiology and cardiology," *Radiation Measurements*, 2011, vol. 46, n° 11, 1324–1329.

[3]Loy Rodas N., Barrera F., Padoy N., "See It with Your Own Eyes: Markerless Mobile Augmented Reality for Radiation Awareness in the Hybrid Room," *IEEE Trans. Biomed. Engineering*, 2017, 64(2), 429–440.

example, risk simulation can be used to optimize the positioning of the imaging device to minimize the dose received by the patient and staff while preserving the visibility of the observed anatomy in the intraoperative image.[4] By combining this approach with accurate detection of 3D positions of the body parts of personnel[5] and with automated recognition of the various gestures and procedural steps[6] it would be possible to compute statistics on the doses received for each body part and for each type of activity over long periods. This would provide objective information that could be used by radiation safety professionals to assess risks, monitor long-term exposure, and optimize surgical processes.

## Analysis of Activities in Laparoscopic Surgery

The recognition of operating room activities irrespective of whether they are surgical gestures performed on patients or peripheral activities has many applications beyond the objective analysis of radiation exposure mentioned at the end of the previous section. Recognition is at the core of the operating room control tower because it is this technology that is essential for the development of assistance tools that can be reactive to the operating context. Laparoscopic surgery is the preferred type of surgery when it comes to studying recognition of surgical activities because the videos generated by cameras are easily accessible. To take advantage of the large numbers of videos generated in the operating room their intraoperative or postoperative analysis must, however, be automated.

Our objective is to exploit these videos using machine learning techniques to model and recognize certain surgical activities in real time including surgical steps and interactions between the tools and the anatomy.[7] Another objective is to predict additional relevant information such as the remaining time of an intervention.[8] We focused our study on cholecystectomy, a frequent and well-standardized surgery. To do this we built a dataset containing 120 laparoscopic videos manually annotated

---

[4]Loy Rodas N., Bert J., Visvikis D., de Mathelin M., Padoy N., "Pose optimization of a C-arm imaging device to reduce intraoperative radiation exposure of staff and patients during interventional procedures," *ICRA*, 2017, 4200–4207.

[5]Kadkhodamohammadi A., Gangi A., de Mathelin M., Padoy N., "Articulated clinician detection using 3D pictorial structures on RGB-D data," *Medical Image Analysis*, 2017, 35, 215–224.

[6]Twinanda A.P., "Vision-based approaches for surgical activity recognition using laparoscopic and RGBD videos," Ph.D. thesis, Strasbourg University, 2017.

[7]Twinanda A.P., Shehata S., Mutter D., Marescaux J., de Mathelin M., Padoy N., "EndoNet: A Deep Architecture for Recognition Tasks on Laparoscopic Videos," *IEEE Trans. Med. Imaging*, 2017, 36(1), 86–97.

[8]Aksamentov I., Twinanda A.P., Mutter D., Marescaux J., Padoy N., "Deep Neural Networks Predict Remaining Surgery Duration from Cholecystectomy Videos," *MICCAI* (2), 2017, 586–593.

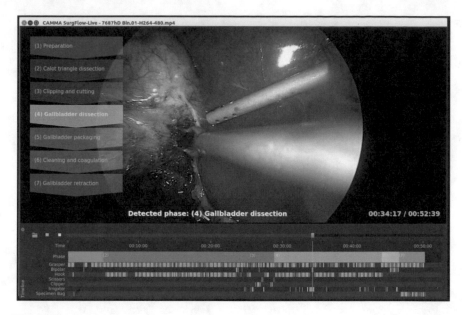

**Fig. 3** Prototype used for the recognition of surgical activities such as surgical steps from laparoscopic videos

with information describing the operating steps and tools used. Then, we proposed and trained deep and recurrent neural networks on this database making it possible to recognize this same type of information on new videos in real time. A recognition rate exceeding 90% suggests the possibility of integrating this type of approach into an operating room control tower making it possible to create context-sensitive user interfaces, facilitate report writing by automatically integrating relevant information and index videos to enable their navigation, comparison, and analysis (e.g., during training and accreditation sessions). Such a tool is illustrated in Fig. 3.

For such methods to have an impact in hospitals it will still be necessary to show that they can be generalized to other types of common surgeries and practices since their robustness to the wide range of potential activities is essential to their use. Demonstrating that they can scale up will be a challenge when it comes to the fully supervised methods currently used because annotating data is time-consuming and very costly. It will therefore be necessary to develop new semi-supervised methods that require little manual intervention but are capable of exploiting the large amounts of unannotated surgical data available to increase their generalizability, accuracy, and robustness.

# High-Dimensional Statistical Learning and Its Application to Oncological Diagnosis by Radiomics

Charles Bouveyron

## Introduction: Learning, Curse, and Blessing of Dimensionality

Statistical learning is today playing an increasing role in many scientific fields as varied as medicine, imagery, biology, and astronomy. Scientific advances in recent years have significantly increased measurement and calculation capabilities, and it is now difficult for a human operator to process such data exhaustively in a timely manner. In particular, many medical specialties such as medical imaging, radiology, and genomics have benefited in recent decades from major technological developments. In some instances these developments have led specialists in these fields to rethink their data practice.

Statistical learning must be seen as a subdiscipline of what is now commonly referred to as artificial intelligence (AI) and is proposed to take over from the human expert to model and synthesize such complex data to assist practitioners in decision-making. Supervised classification (or discriminant analysis) in medical applications is probably the most commonly used learning method for diagnosis or prognosis related to pathologies. Nevertheless, some practical situations correspond to theoretical problems that are not fully solved. For example, the classification of very high–dimensional data or the classification of correlated data are problems that are particularly prevalent in image analysis and biology. Although current solutions are already very advanced, they require further research.

In particular, the high dimensionality of data (large numbers of variables) poses a set of problems for classical multivariate statistics usually characterized as the "curse of dimensionality." Problems with high-dimensional data include numerical problems, inference problems, and problems related to estimator bias. It has therefore

C. Bouveyron (✉)
Université Côte d'Azur, Laboratoire J.A. Dieudonné, UMR CNRS 7351, Nice, France
e-mail: charles.bouveyron@univ-cotedazur.fr

INRIA, Maasai team, Valbonne, France

© Springer Nature Switzerland AG 2020
B. Nordlinger et al. (eds.), *Healthcare and Artificial Intelligence*,
https://doi.org/10.1007/978-3-030-32161-1_17

been necessary in recent years to develop methods to overcome these problems. This chapter will explore problems and hopes (blessings) that relate to the high dimensionality of data. It also investigates some recent statistical learning methods that make better analysis and understanding of medical data possible.

## Curse and Blessing of Dimensionality

If there is one expression that can be classically associated with high-dimensional data it is the "curse of dimensionality" first introduced by Richard Bellman in the late 1950s. Bellman used this phrase in the preface to his book *Dynamic Programming* to summarize all the difficulties posed by high-dimensional spaces. Such spaces often have surprising properties, and it is generally difficult to extrapolate the properties of what is known from 2D or 3D spaces to spaces of higher dimensions. A simple way to observe this is to look at the volume of the hypersphere[1] unit according to the size of the space. This volume is given by the formula $V(p) = \pi^{(p/2)}/\Gamma(p/2 + 1)$. Figure 1 facilitates visualizing the way in which this function evolves with respect to dimension $p$ of the space. It is clear that the volume of the hypersphere beyond dimension five tends toward zero very quickly, which is clearly counterintuitive. Learning in such spaces from a statistical point of view is confronted with numerical problems related to overparameterization[2] or problems of bias in estimation.

On the other hand, high-dimensional spaces have characteristics that bring a little hope and can be seen as a blessing in relation to the abovementioned problems. The phenomenon of "empty space" highlighted in the late 1970s reflects the fact that high-dimensional spaces are mainly empty and that high-dimensional data are

**Fig. 1** Evolution of the volume of the hypersphere unit as a function of the size of the space

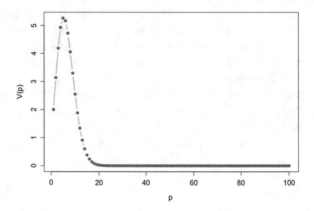

---

[1]The hypersphere is the generalization used for the ordinary sphere in spaces that have more than three dimensions.

[2]Some learning methods have a number of parameters that increase with the size of the space, which can be problematic in high dimensions.

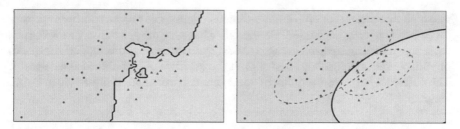

**Fig. 2** Classification boundaries of a discriminative classifier (left) and a generative classifier (right)

grouped into small subspaces. This can clearly be an advantage when wanting to discriminate between classes of individuals, but numerical problems and estimation bias must be overcome for this to happen. Figure 2 shows that an "oracle" classifier benefits from this phenomenon, while the classifier learned from the data degrades the performance it obtains in small dimensions. The hope of exploiting the phenomenon of empty space in classification therefore depends on the ability to effectively solve the statistical inference problem.

## *Common Approaches to High-Dimensional Learning*

The usual approaches used to overcome problems posed by high-dimensional data are dimensionality reduction, regularization, and the use of parsimonious models. Dimensionality reduction is certainly the oldest and most useful approach in practice.[3] It is the most direct way of countering the problem of high dimensionality, but it has the disadvantage of potentially generating a loss of discriminative information. Regularization addresses numerical problems (particularly, those due to the high collinearity of variables). However, these adjustment techniques can be difficult to set up. Finally, parsimonious approaches oblige models to reduce their level of parameterization, even if it means sometimes making strong assumptions such as the conditional independence of variables.[4]

## Recent Advances in High-Dimensional Learning

Recent methods used to classify high-dimensional data make full use of the phenomenon of empty space. On the one hand, of the discriminative methods (i.e., those with the sole purpose of building a classification function) kernel methods (vector machine support), and convolutional neural networks do not hesitate to project data

---

[3]Two vectors $u$ and $v$ are said to be collinear if there is a scalar $\lambda$ such that $v = \lambda u$.

[4]Some models assume that the covariance matrix of each class is diagonal.

into high-dimensional or even infinite-dimensional spaces using a non-linear projector to facilitate class separation. On the other hand, of the generative methods (i.e., those that model classes and derive a classification rule from this model) subspaces or variable selection methods best exploit the qualities of high-dimensional spaces. The difference between discriminative and generative methods is illustrated in Fig. 2.

## Classification in Subspaces

The oldest work in this context is the seminal work of R.A. Fisher who introduced linear discriminant analysis (LDA) in 1936. It later became known as Fisher[5] discriminant analysis. The objective of LDA is to find a low-dimensional subspace that best discriminates between classes. Even though LDA can suffer from the collinearity of variables, it remains a standard method that mostly provides very satisfactory results. Two of the most recent and commonly used methods, partial least square discriminant analysis (PLSDA)[6] and high-dimensional discriminant analysis (HDDA),[7] assume that data live in subspaces. PLSDA looks for latent representations of the data and the variable to be predicted such that the covariance between the two is maximum. It is a method widely used in disciplines such as genomics or metabolomics. HDDA is based on statistical modeling that assumes that the data of each class live in different subspaces and with different intrinsic dimensions. Thus HDDA can be used

**Fig. 3** Class modeling in specific subspaces

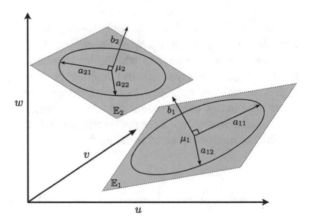

[5]Fisher R.A., "The use of multiple measurements in taxonomic problems," *Annals of Eugenics*, 1936, vol. 7, 179–188.

[6]Barker M., Rayens W., "Partial least squares for discrimination," *Journal of Chemometrics*, 2003, vol. 17(3), 166–173.

[7]Bouveyron C., Girard S., Schmid C., "High-Dimensional Data Clustering," *Computational Statistics and Data Analysis*, 2007, vol. 52(1), 502–519.

to finely fit the data and provide a high-performance classifier. Figure 3 illustrates the principle of modeling in subspaces specific to classes.[8]

## Classification by Variable Selection

Variable selection was also explored at an early stage to overcome the problem of high dimensions while maintaining the advantage of interpretation over original variables. The Fisher criterion can also be used in this context, and the Wilks' Lambda can be used to construct statistical tests to decide the usefulness of a variable. Unfortunately, these approaches quickly encountered the combinatorics of exploring subsets of many variables. It was not until the early 2000s that the new approach of variable selection by Lasso sparsity emerged. Lasso approaches select variables by adding to the objective-learning function.

However, the Lasso approach requires defining the level of parsimony usually done by cross-validation. One of the so-called sparser methods of classification is sparse discriminant analysis (SDA). Proposed by Witten and Tibshirani[9] it introduces parsimony into the LDA method through an $\ell_1$ penalty.

## Selection of Variables in Bayesian Parsimonious Classification

Recently, Mattei et al.[10] introduced in the context of principal component analysis (PCA) a parsimony structured a priori as Bayesian.[11] The resulting method called globally sparse probabilistic PCA (gsPPCA) reduces the dimensionality of a dataset while selecting variables that can be used to describe the data. This approach has also been extended to the classification framework by transferring the parsimony structured a priori as Bayesian within HDDA. Thus the resulting HDDA sparse method (sHDDA)[12] makes it possible to select the variables necessary to model each class independently. To do this sHDDA assumes that each class is distributed according to a normal distribution:

---

[8]Readers wanting more details on this type of approach should consult Bouveyron C., Brunet-Saumard C., "Model-based clustering of high-dimensional data: A review," *Computational Statistics and Data Analysis*, 2014, vol. 71, pp. 52–78.

[9]Witten D., Tibshirani R., "Penalized classification using Fisher's linear discriminant analysis," *Journal of the Royal Statistical Society: Series B (Statistical Methodology)*, 2011, vol. 73(5), 753–772.

[10]Mattei P.-A., Bouveyron C., Latouche P., *Bayesian Variable Selection for Globally Sparse Probabilistic PCA*, Preprint HAL No. 01310409, Paris Descartes University, 2016.

[11]Some parameters of the model are then seen as random variables with their own a priori distribution.

[12]Orlhac F., Mattei P.-A., Bouveyron C., Ayache N., *Class-specific Variable Selection in High-dimensional Discriminant Analysis through Bayesian Sparsity*, Preprint HAL No. 01811514, Côte d'Azur University, 2018.

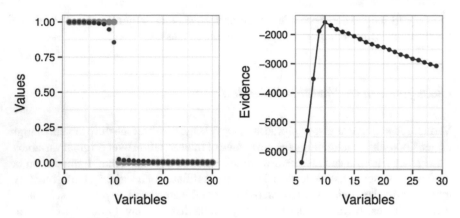

**Fig. 4** Variable selection operated by sHDDA for a class

$$X|Z = k \sim N(\mu_k, \Sigma_k) = V_k S_k V_k^t + b_k I_p$$

where $V_k = \mathrm{diag}(v_1, \ldots, v_k, \ldots, v_p)$, a binary diagonal matrix, indicating whether or not each of the $p$ variables can be used for modeling class $k$. It should be noted that, unlike Lasso approaches, gsPPCA and sHDDA do not use cross-validation to determine the number of relevant variables because this parameter is inherent in modeling. Indeed, gsPPCA and sHDDA optimize the marginal likelihood of a model being selected with respect to $v_k$ variables over a range of models. Figure 4 illustrates the choice of the number of relevant variables for one of the classes.

## Application of Radiomics to Oncological Diagnosis

Radiomics is an emerging technique used in medical research that consists of extracting tumor characteristics from medical images such as magnetic resonance imaging (MRI), computed tomography (CT), or positron emission tomography (PET) scans. Such characteristics describe tumor heterogeneity, shape, and texture. The number of variables extracted can vary depending on the technology used from a few dozen to several hundred variables. Training a high-performance classifier is complicated by the fact that most studies include fewer than 100 patients. The ratio between number of patients and number of variables does not then favor statistical estimate. Classification methods such as sHDDA inspire us with hope to effectively discriminate the subtype of lesion (which could reduce the number of biopsies required) while selecting the relevant variables needed to describe each subtype and thus providing a better understanding of the various subtypes.'

A recent study by Orlhac et al. illustrates the possibilities of using radiomics to predict the histological subtype in breast cancer.[13] In this study the authors investigated a cohort of 26 breast cancer patients treated at the Centre Antoine Lacassagne in Nice. They found that 7 of the 26 patients had a triple-negative lesion, a particularly aggressive type of tumor. PET images were available for all patients and 43 radiomic variables were extracted using LIFEx software. Analysis of the operating room using a mass spectrometer identified 1500 metabolites found in the Human Metabolome Database. After showing that most of the 43 radiomic variables correlated highly with at least 50 metabolites the authors compared the suitability of five high-dimension classification methods to predict the histological subtype (triple-negative against the rest) on radiomic variables and then on metabolomic variables. Figure 5 shows the classification results (25-fold cross-validation). Youden's score ($Y$ = sensitivity + specificity − 1) was used to evaluate performance. It should be remembered that a perfect classifier will have a Youden's score equal to 1. It should be noted that the HDDA and sHDDA methods (which select variables) are particularly efficient and that the best results are obtained from radiomic variables. Figure 6 also shows

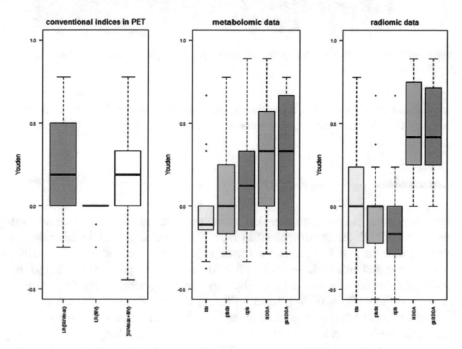

**Fig. 5** Classification performance (Youden score) of various methods for triple-negative prediction Courtesy Orlhac et al. (2018)

[13]Orlhac F., Humbert O., Pourcher T., Jing L., Guigonis J.-M., Darcourt J., Bouveyron C., Ayache N., "Statistical analysis of PET radiomic features and metabolomic data: Prediction of triple-negative breast cancer," SNMMI 2018 Annual Meeting, *Journal of Nuclear Medicine*, 2018, vol. 59, p. 1755.

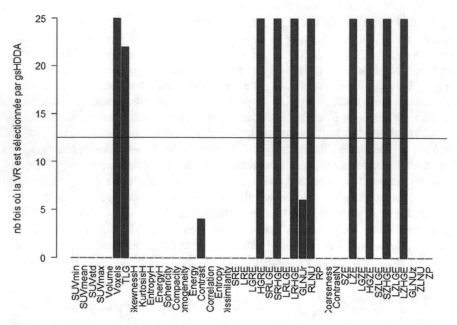

**Fig. 6** Radiomic variables selected by the sHDDA method for triple-negative prediction. Courtesy Orlhac et al. (2018)

variables selected by sHDDA according to the number of replications. It should also be noted that the selection is particularly stable despite the low amount of data.

## Conclusion

This chapter has presented an overview of the problems and solutions that are part and parcel of high-dimensional classification. The research carried out in statistical learning over the past 15 years has led to significant progress and made it possible to overcome particularly difficult classification tasks. Such progress has led to the development of advanced tools that can be implemented to achieve significant results in medical fields like oncology based on recent technologies such as radiomics or metabolomics. Data processing could make it possible in the medium term to predict histological subtypes of lesions without the need for a biopsy. A longer term objective would be to use such technologies to predict treatment response during the first few visits of a patient and thus avoid waiting one or more treatment cycles to observe such a response. Statistical learning methods therefore have an important role to play in the exploitation of "omics" data for medical use.

# Mathematical Modeling of Tumors

## A Key Role in the Coming Years?

Thierry Colin

Mathematical modeling and scientific computing are part of the general scientific landscape and universally used in almost all industrial sectors. Car manufacturers use it to optimize their vehicles. In aeronautics, models and calculations are used to design aircraft. In energy, calculations can be used to explore extreme regimes (e.g., by simulating an accident in a nuclear power plant or a dam failure) that cannot of course be reached experimentally. Calculation can also be used to explain complex phenomena or to predict the future. This is the case in climatology. Mathematical models have been used in finance for a very long time, and it has recently become possible to simulate crowd movements or to introduce models that can be used in the social sciences. The usefulness of such numerical simulations is well proven, and scientific computing has now been expanding for quite some while. Mathematical modeling is mature and based on a number of tools developed over the centuries. Such development mostly came about as a result of interaction with the physical sciences and because mathematicians up to the 19th century were almost always also physical and sometimes philosophical scientists. The emergence of computers has led to impressive development of the possibilities offered by modeling and has led to an increase in knowledge because more researchers have been working on it. The Second World War also played a key role in triggering this process.[1] Currently, the production of data and the algorithms associated with the processing of such data only accentuate this trend. The complexity of the phenomena that can be modeled is increasing: it is no longer a problem to try and calculate in an industrial context the icing and deicing phases of an aircraft in unsteady flight, the deformation of the landing gear as an aircraft touches down, the behavior of an offshore wind turbine, or the effect of a tsunami on a shore. Prediction, risk calculation, multiphysical modeling, macromolecule modeling, composite material behavior—everything seems

T. Colin (✉)
Radiomics Business Area, SOPHiA GENETICS, Bordeaux, France
e-mail: tcolin@sophiagenetics.com

[1] Dahan Dalmedico A., "The Rise of Applied Mathematics in the United States: The Impact of the Second World War," *Review of the History of Mathematics*, 2 (1996), 149–213.

© Springer Nature Switzerland AG 2020
B. Nordlinger et al. (eds.), *Healthcare and Artificial Intelligence*,
https://doi.org/10.1007/978-3-030-32161-1_18

accessible to modeling in the physical and chemical sciences. No longer is it deemed absurd to try to model and predict climate with tools that accurately describe ocean movements or atmospheric evolution. It must be said that the predictive power of modeling is still largely untapped in the life sciences, medicine, and more particularly oncology.

The purpose of this chapter is to describe everything that is needed to see what can be done with oncology modeling tools by combining modeling objects, data, data processing, and numerical simulation algorithms.

## Modeling Approach and Obstacles in Oncology

Modern scientific computing used, for example, to digitally simulate the behavior of a tire on a wet road involves a number of steps. Daily practice in scientific or industrial activities shows that different steps are often intertwined because many academic or commercial computation codes are available and make it possible for some of them to be bypassed. Nevertheless, for the purposes of understanding the process and analyzing what can be done in oncology we will try and break down the modeling process. The first step involves developing the mathematical model itself. When it comes to considering our tire we will have to be able to describe its mechanical behavior (i.e., an elastic solid). It will also be necessary to be able to model the movement of water (i.e., the movement of a fluid), and because the tire is inflated it will also be necessary to be able to model the movement of a gas. Describing these three states of matter will not be sufficient on their own and it will still be necessary to manage their interactions. How does this work? Let's take the example of a fluid formed by molecules that slide one on top of the other. If we try to describe a fluid in this way (as a set of molecules that slide over each other), we will quickly realize the task is futile. All the computers in the world will not be enough to describe what happens in a thimble when you want to calculate ocean movements. This will be so for a long time to come! When we further consider that we should also take into account the shape of the molecules (specific for each fluid) and their position in space the futility we feel becomes even worse. Of course, no computational code is based on these principles thanks to centuries of physics developing the mechanics of continuous media and making it possible to consider a fluid, gas, or solid as a continuous medium (this is the macroscopic image we have of it in everyday life) and not as a pile of discrete elements (molecules or atoms). The mechanics of continuous media will be based on describing the movement of infinitesimal elements small enough to consider the fluid as the union of an infinite number of such elements but large enough to contain a multitude of molecules so that at their scale we no longer see the separate influence of the molecules, but we can still describe the fluid by the interaction of these elements. Such elements will

$$\rho(\partial u + u \cdot u) + p = v\Delta u + F$$
$$\nabla \cdot u = 0$$

$$\rho\left(\partial_t u + u \cdot \nabla u\right) + \nabla p = \nu\Delta u + F$$
$$\nabla \cdot u = 0$$

**Fig. 1** Navier–Stokes equations for an incompressible Newtonian fluid where $u$ is the velocity of the fluid, $p$ is the pressure, $\rho$ is its density, and $F$ the external forces

then be convected by the velocity of the fluid, and friction with neighboring elements will be modeled using the notion of viscosity.[2]

This will allow us to write the equations that govern the movement of all fluids—not that of a particular fluid. That is the great strength of this type of modeling. Such modeling makes it possible to design the mathematical model of the notion of fluid, in general, then to particularize it to a specific fluid, and finally to implement it in a given situation. Once these equations are known, it is then necessary to determine the physical quantities that characterize this fluid such as its density, viscosity, and thermal properties. In Fig. 1 we give the so-called Navier–Stokes equations that govern the evolution of all incompressible Newtonian viscous fluids.

Does this mean that we know how to model all situations in mechanics? No, of course not! Moreover, for complex fluids the equivalent of the equations in Fig. 1 is only partially known. Furthermore, it is necessary to specify how these equations are obtained. It is a question of writing generic laws that reflect the conservation of mass, the conservation of energy, and the conservation of linear momentum. The invariance conditions of certain geometric and/or physical indicators may also be taken into account. If we are interested in phenomena that involve electromagnetic phenomena (microwave heating, laser machining, etc.), we will have to add to the previous models the Maxwell equations that govern electromagnetism. If we are in a framework of reactive flows (combustion or chemical reaction), then it will be necessary to model these phenomena (Arrhenius law, mass action law). There are many possibilities to do so. This approach is made globally possible because after centuries of effort we understand the fundamental laws of physics, at least on the macroscopic scale. The rest of the modeling process will consist in particularizing the model to basically configure it to a situation and to its components. In a physical situation we can make measurements and experiments. This will of course not be possible in medicine since we know very well that in vitro experiments cannot be transposed in vivo and that extrapolation from animals to humans is impossible from a quantitative point of view. This parameterization problem is critical. The next step in our computational process is discretization that consists in transforming continuous equations (such as in Fig. 1) into discrete equations that can be interpreted by a computer. Fortunately for us the mathematical techniques developed since the middle of the 20th century are independent of the field of application and are universal. Finally, to be able to apply these discretization techniques it is necessary to have "meshed" the geometry

---

[2]Many books deal with the process of mechanical modeling. A good example is Caltagirone J.P., *Physics of Continuous Flow*, Springer (Mathematics and Applications Series), 2013.

of the organ or the calculation zone (i.e., to have "pixelated" the organ even though the precise calculations are done on objects more complex than a pixel). We can use MMG software to get an idea of what mesh size[3] is all about.

## Tumor Growth Modeling

Cancer is a multiscale disease in the sense that phenomena occurring on very different scales of space and time are intertwined. Cancer that is seen as a DNA disease involves variants of certain genes that deregulate proper functioning of a cell. From the molecular level (i.e., the nanometer level) we move to the cellular level (the micrometer level). The functioning of this abnormal cell locally disrupts the organization of tissue by modifying the microenvironment (millimeter scale), particularly angiogenesis (manufacture of new blood vessels), then altering the functioning of the organ (decimeter scale), and finally the metastases spread the disease throughout the whole body (therefore at a scale of about 1 m). So nine orders of magnitude are involved. The same is true at the temporal level from activation of a signaling pathway to metastatic dissemination a few months later. It is therefore of course impossible to model tumor progression from the gene to the organ as this would be unrealistic. Imagine then how unrealistic it would be to model fluid flow (or fluid mixture) by calculating the friction of molecules on each other! We will therefore use macroscopic approaches to describe tumor growth. It is at this level that we encounter the first major difference from physical modeling. We do not know any fundamental laws of biology or medicine from which we could construct hierarchies of models capable of describing living tissues and organisms in a generic way whether in a nominal regime (healthy organism) or in a pathological regime. This is particularly true in oncology, an area where the cause of disease is unknown, even though we understand some mechanisms and some risk factors.

Our strategy will be to overcome this major obstacle by designing models that are not derived from a "source model" representing a "general" tumor but on the contrary by developing a series of models each adapted to a tumor type based on available data. This approach has the advantage of pragmatism despite being less satisfactory from an intellectual point of view. We will describe some of the ways in which this can be done to achieve promising results. To do this we will rely on the knowledge and data available in oncology. In the same way that we work with infinitesimal elements of matter in the mechanics of continuous media we will work with infinitesimal elements of tissue. We will describe tissue by quantifying the density of cells per unit volume at each point in space.

The difficulty will then be to quantify the extent to which this density evolves over time. It is extremely tempting to put a lot of biological information into it, something

---

[3]MMG platform: https://www.mmgtools.org.

the author of this chapter has done.[4] This results in systems of great mathematical complexity capable of effectively accounting for complex biological phenomena (in this case the response to experimental treatments). On the other hand, the use of such systems in a clinical context remains illusory because they are very far removed from real data. A detour to the available data is required.

## Available Data in Clinical Oncology

Patients diagnosed with cancer will undergo a number of tests that refine the diagnosis and lead the healthcare team to choose the most appropriate treatment. Biopsy is a part of such treatments and consists in taking a tissue sample to qualify the disease at the level of the type of cells involved. Alternatively, histological examination can be done on a tumor resected by the surgeon. The description provided by the pathologist will make first classification of the tumor possible. Thus, a primary lung tumor can be clearly differentiated from a metastasis of a distant cancer. Tissues are increasingly being analyzed at the genomic level. The analysis of data produced by new-generation sequencers enables rapid and accurate detection of gene alterations that are known to play an active role in development of the disease. Thus, with lung cancer at least 20 genes are almost systematically tested on tissues obtained during biopsy or surgery. A number of alterations not necessarily present in all tumor cells are commonly highlighted. We are therefore dealing with pluriclonal diseases in which several types of tumor cells have different behaviors or resistance to treatment. This is another point that will have to be taken into account in the model. However, the main source of data remains imagery. Medical imaging plays a key role in oncology and is involved at all levels of the patient's care journey from diagnosis, assessment of the extension of the disease, to follow-up of the patient during treatment, and finally to the monitoring phase. Imaging can provide morphological information about the tumor such as shape, size, density, and topography. This is mainly achieved using computed tomography (CT) scans (in short, scanners), ultrasound imaging (ultrasound), and basic magnetic resonance imaging (MRI) sequences. Imaging can also provide functional information such as perfusion MRI and positron emission tomography (PET) imaging. Imaging has a role to play in monitoring disease progression (for diagnosis and relapse detection). It also plays a quantification role to assess the quality of the response to treatment to decide whether or not to modify the management of a patient. Finally, imaging also plays a guiding role for a whole series of minimally invasive procedures such as percutaneous removal of lesions by radiofrequency, cryoablation, microwaves, and focused ultrasound. It also plays such a role for surgery and radiotherapy. Our description would be incomplete without mentioning the massive

---

[4]Billy F., Ribba B., Saut O., Morre-Trouilhet H., Colin Th., Bresch D., Boissel J.-P., Grenier E., Flandrois J.-P., "A pharmacologically-based multiscale mathematical model of angiogenesis, and its use in analysing the efficacy of a new anti-cancer treatment strategy," *Journal of Theoretical Biology*, October 2009, vol. 260, issue 4, 545–562.

improvement in the quality and accuracy of images in recent years. Pixels are now submillimetric in scanner imaging. In MRI the order of magnitude is 1.5 mm for T1 sequences. PET imaging is a little coarser with 5-mm pixels. Functional sequences in MRI are very variable depending on the target organ, the machine, the operator, etc. Each 3D image therefore represents a significant amount of information both quantitatively and literally. It should be kept in mind that a thorax–abdomen–pelvis scanner will "weigh" at least 500 MB. Patients during their care journey will therefore benefit from numerous imaging examinations. This mass of information is still very largely untapped in terms of data mining. There are several reasons for this: data are widely dispersed in hospitals; raw images are complicated to interpret (e.g., a scanner will give a density of tissue that must be linked to biology and MRI returns a signal with better contrasts and more precision but is even more complicated to quantify); and, finally, since such data are obviously specific to each patient it must therefore be possible to link them to the patient's clinical history.

The last point concerns quantification of the effects of treatments. The "usual" criterion for response to treatment is the response evaluation criteria in solid tumors (RECIST), which simply consists in measuring the largest diameter of the tumor and monitoring its evolution from one examination to another. A variation between 20% more and 30% less stipulates the status of the disease such as "in progression," "partial response" of the patient, or "stable" if the variation falls between these two values. Because of its simplicity this criterion has made it possible to standardize procedures and its effectiveness for radiotherapy and chemotherapy has been proven. Chemotherapy treatment response rates such as the objective response rate (ORR) are generally correlated with overall survival (OS). Nevertheless, the effectiveness of treatments (drug and interventional) has brought about considerably increased survival times despite increasingly complex clinical situations and imaging data that are too subtle to be interpreted by the human eye. In addition, new anticancer treatments (targeted therapies, antiangiogenic therapies, immunotherapies) do not only directly kill tumor cells but also attack tumor function by trying to inhibit the signaling pathways that control cell proliferation, by destroying tumor neovascularization, or by tagging the tumor for the immune system to destroy it (immune checkpoint inhibitors). Evaluating the effectiveness of these imaging treatments for oncology is currently a major challenge in radiology. For example, there is a need for immunotherapy to distinguish pseudoprogressions from real progressions as quickly as possible. The evolutionary patterns of diseases in this context are very largely unknown. All these elements must be taken into account at the model level.

## Some Ideas for Modeling and Using Data in Oncology: General Principles

The first step will be to build a system of equations capable of describing tumor growth (equivalent to the Navier–Stokes equations in Fig. 1) bearing in mind that the complexity of such a system will have to be controlled if we want to move toward client-oriented applications. We will therefore resist the temptation to describe the cells one by one, the mutations present, the interactions, etc., but instead we will try to "copy" the mechanics of continuous media and give global formulations. This was the approach chosen by Ambrosi and Preziosi[5] who, for example, adapted fluid–mixture models by transforming them into cell–mixture models. A decision now needs to be made regarding how many different kinds of cells should be considered based on biological data. The answer is complex and pushes us toward the realization that we will need one model per tumor type and perhaps even several per tumor type depending on the data that will be available. In any case it seems reasonable to use "healthy" cells, proliferative cells, and quiescent tumor cells. It is at this level that several populations of proliferating cells (several clones) may be introduced that may or may not resist certain treatments. This is what has been done in the modeling of gastrointestinal stromal tumors (GISTs) to describe resistance to targeted therapies.[6] After defining the number of populations of proliferating cells, we need to define spatial spread (extension) and proliferation itself, the two drivers of tumor progression. When dealing with spatial extension of an infiltrating tumor, we will favor models based on diffusion equations such as those historically used by K. R. Swanson in his work on gliomas[7] and extended by Konukoglu et al.[8] However, when dealing with pulmonary metastases or meningiomas, we will prefer mechanical models. This is because such models describe the fact that it is cell proliferation that increases pressure by locally increasing volume and creates a displacement in the opposite direction to the pressure gradient. This description is well suited to compact tumors that present themselves as growing masses and are therefore quite different from the infiltrating tumors just described. The last step is by far the most delicate and involves choosing a mode of proliferation. Although epidemiologists, ecologists, and mathematicians have long studied these population dynamics models, no single model has managed to achieve consensus. Indeed, we are talking here about *local* growth models that can be observed over a limited timescale and can therefore describe the rate of local cellular proliferation in space for the duration of the disease. It will then be necessary to calculate the total volume of the tumor and its evolution over time to obtain an estimate of the overall behavior. Thus, an exponential growth model whose rate depends on space might well discern linear growth in tumor volume. Conversely, a Gompertz-type growth model (i.e., with a priori saturation of the total volume) might well discern linear, even exponential,

---

[5] Ambrosi D., Preziosi L., "On the closure of mass balance models for tumor growth," *Math. Models Method Appl. Sci.*, 2002, 12, 737–754.

[6] Lefebvre G., Cornelis F., Cumsille P., Colin Th., Poignard C., Saut O., "Spatial modeling of tumor drug resistance: The case of GIST liver metastasis," *Mathematical Medicine & Biology*, March 2016.

[7] Swanson K.R., Bridge C., Murray J.D., Alvord E.C., "Virtual and real brain tumors: Using mathematical modeling to quantify glioma growth and invasion," *J Neuro Sci*, 2003, 216, 1–10.

[8] Konukoglu E., Clatz O., Bondiau P.Y., Delingette H., Ayache N.
"Extrapolating glioma invasion margin in brain magnetic resonance images: Suggesting new irradiation margins," *Medical Image Analysis*, 2010, 14, 111–125.

growth at the spatiotemporal scale of the study! Nevertheless, description of such a growth rate may well make it possible to introduce fine-modeling elements such as angiogenesis and immune system response.

## Two Examples of Tumor Growth: Meningiomas and Lung Metastases

Once you have built a model along the lines described above, you have to ask yourself whether such a model can be used to help a doctor better manage the patient in much the same way as a digital model makes safer aircraft possible. The monitoring of meningiomas is a good starting point. Meningiomas are the most common primary brain tumors. They develop from the inner layer of the skull (the arachnoid) and are benign tumors (i.e., not cancers), but their mechanical effect on the brain causes neurological effects. The treatments are neurosurgery and radiotherapy. For asymptomatic meningiomas the strategy is often to monitor growth and intervene only when symptoms appear or growth accelerates. It is clear that the term "accelerating growth" is quite subjective. Having a tool to simulate and predict growth is indeed an asset for the neurosurgeon. Construction of a meningioma model does not present any particular difficulties; however, it remains an obstacle to particularize this model for each patient. We do not currently know how to use an initial image of the disease (e.g., an MRI of the skull) to be able to simulate progression of the disease because there is a lack of quantitative data. Such a difficulty can be overcome by looking at the radiologist's way of working. The radiologist as soon as he can compares the examination that has just been done with a previous examination to evaluate the changes. We will adopt this strategy but in a quantitative way. By considering two successive MRIs of the same patient we will try and ascertain the values of parameters to put in the models. Therefore, by simulating tumor evolution using the first MRI as the starting point the result of the simulation best represents what we see on the second image. Once you have determined these parameters (the opposite problem has been solved), then evolution of the tumor can be simulated over time (i.e., tumor evolution can be predicted accurately and individually). Such a 3D simulation of a meningioma over a two-year period can be found online (see screenshot in Fig. 2).[9]

The same strategy can be developed for the growth of pulmonary metastases without treatment for oligometastatic cases. In the same way (i.e., relying on two consecutive scanner examinations) we will be able to reconstruct the evolution of

---

[9]https://www.youtube.com/watch?v=l6XvWZXQNlg Joint work between H. Loiseau (CHU de Bordeaux), G. Kantor (Institut Bergonié), O. Saut (INRIA), and V. Piannet (SOPHiA GENETICS).

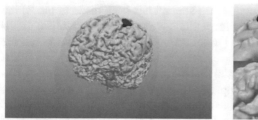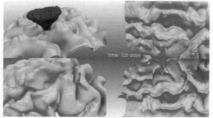

**Fig. 2** Simulation of the growth of a meningioma. (*left*) Location of the meningioma at the initial moment. (*right*) Evolution after 725 days, shape of the meningioma, and deformation of the cerebral parenchyma due to the meningioma

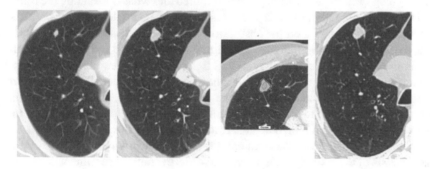

T=0 days          T=294 days.    Prediction at T=405 days.  CT-scan at T=405 days

**Fig. 3** Calculating the evolution of an isolated pulmonary metastasis. The first two scans (at $T = 0$ day and $T = 294$ days) are used to produce a simulation at time $T = 405$ days. The software then provides the shape of the tumor shown in *blue* on the image. This contour can then be compared with what is observed on the scan (*right*) performed at $T = 405$ days

pulmonary metastasis and arrive at a prediction. A 3D simulation of lung metastasis can be found online (see Fig. 3).[10]

## Example Response to Treatment: Kidney Cancers Treated with Antiangiogens

The challenge in oncology is to understand the response to treatment so that each patient can be given the most appropriate treatment; hence the need to be able to

---

[10]https://www.youtube.com/watch?v=A2lBIdl-KwQ& Joint work between J. Palussière (Institut Bergonié), F. Cornelis (Tenon Hospital, AP-HP), O. Saut and M. Martin (INRIA), and V. Piannet (SOPHiA GENETICS).

model the effect of a treatment. Of course, no attempt has been made to model the effect of a treatment at the microscopic level since we are targeting clinical applications. Nevertheless, the tumor growth model adopted must take into account the treatment envisioned. Thus, to describe the effect of antiangiogenic treatments aimed at reducing tumor angiogenesis it is essential that the model contain a module describing such angiogenesis. However, the complexity of such a module must be such that parameterization from imaging data is possible. This begs the question of how to estimate the effects of antiangiogenic drugs on imaging data. Infusion sequences of examinations using imaging technology makes it possible to obtain information on the vascularization of tissue, but this information remains very difficult to quantify and use in a model. The idea then is to search the image for indirect elements. This requires going back to the way images are acquired and what is meant by measured signal strength. Let's take the case of scanners because it is simpler than that of MRIs. X-ray tomography is based on the absorption of X-rays by tissues. The denser the fabric, the higher the absorption rate. The signal thus recovered is therefore directly "proportional" to the density of the fabric. High intensities (i.e., the densest parts) when it comes to representation appear brightest on the screen and the less dense are therefore dark. When we study a scanner image of a tumor, we can clearly see that the densest areas correspond to areas of high cellularity and therefore to portions of the tumor where proliferation is significant. At the other end of the spectrum dark areas correspond to less dense portions that can be linked to necrotic parts of the tumor. Thus, analysis of the texture of the image and of its evolution over time will give us functional information. Such textural analysis will allow us to understand the effect of a treatment by going beyond the notion of tumor size. The difficulty of course is having algorithms capable of extracting this texture information and transforming it into biologically efficient information. The key once again is to model the spatial evolution of the disease by associating a partially "necrotic" cellular compartment with the dark areas of the image and a "proliferating" compartment with bright areas. An example is shown in Fig. 4 (joint work between F. Cornelis (CHU de Bordeaux) and I. Saut and A. Peretti (INRIA).

## Conclusion

Simulation in oncology is still in its infancy and many years of clinical validations lie ahead. Nevertheless, just as scientific computational tools are ubiquitous in science and industry so it is likely to be in medicine in the near future. As the reader may have noted we deliberately avoided referring to any notion of cohort and statistical analysis in this chapter to emphasize the precise customizable aspect of these models. This should not be taken to mean we can do without population-based analysis on these problems. On the contrary, the most effective tools will be those that combine advanced biomechanical modeling techniques with imaging and genomic databases. Although the results presented in this chapter are elegant and seem spectacular, the real revolution will be the next phase that will consist of using both imaging and

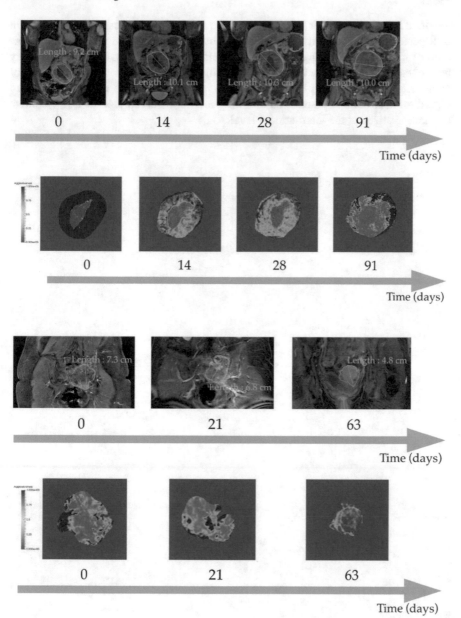

**Fig. 4** Two series of images showing the response of kidney cancer metastases to antiangiogenic treatment. Raw images are on the *top line* of each series and the interpretation of tumor heterogeneity by the software is given on the *lower line* of each series. Proliferation zones are shown in *red* and necrotic zones are shown in *blue*. From the first series we can see that even if the lesion increases slightly its activity (interpreted through texture analysis) decreases significantly despite a proliferation crown possibly remaining. This corresponds to a clinically stable situation. From the second series we can see that even if the size of the lesion decreases sharply there is a concentration of *red* zones. This corresponds to a poor prognosis and a disease that will progress rapidly

genomic data on the tumor to predict tumor progression and response to treatment in a perfectly personalized way. The near future holds out the prospect of a new kind of multiscale modeling in the health field that will consist in integrating very heterogeneous data paving the way for revolutionary approaches for the benefit of patients. A key point will be the appropriation by physicians of these advanced digital tools in clinical practice so that they are not reserved just for a few centers but democratized at the international level.

# Toward an Augmented Radiologist

Mostafa El Hajjam

Some believe the development of increasingly sophisticated image analysis and processing algorithms is likely to lead to the disappearance of the radiologist's profession because they are convinced that the machine will very quickly supplant the eye's abilities and that there will therefore no longer be any need for human intervention to interpret images.

The question about whether artificial intelligence and medical imaging are competing or complementary was the theme of a conference organized on May 2, 2018 at the Collège de France entitled "Medical imaging and automatic learning: Towards artificial intelligence?"

Therefore, questions arise regarding the consequences of the development of artificial intelligence on the radiology profession and how to adapt training to new technologies at a time when the profession is facing a demographic crisis. Fears that machines will replace humans run the risk of leaving students unmotivated and encouraging them to move on to other fields. The consequences are especially damaging at a time when the decline in the demography of radiologists in France threatens to disrupt the healthcare system.

Currently, a hospital cannot function without a radiologist. More than 75% of the 10 million patients admitted annually to Assistance Publique des Hôpitaux de Paris (AP-HP) have an imaging examination. This number is constantly increasing because such examinations lie at the heart of diagnoses.

The vast majority of radiologists are convinced of the help that new technologies and artificial intelligence can bring to their profession, but do not think radiologists as such will be replaced entirely. Artificial intelligence specialists who announce the replacement of radiologists by machines broadcast by the media would do well to realize that a sick human being cannot be reduced to a number of pixels.

---

M. El Hajjam (✉)
Department of Imaging and Interventional Radiology, Ambroise Paré Hospital,
Boulogne-Billancourt, France
e-mail: elhajjam.mostafa@wanadoo.fr

© Springer Nature Switzerland AG 2020
B. Nordlinger et al. (eds.), *Healthcare and Artificial Intelligence*,
https://doi.org/10.1007/978-3-030-32161-1_19

The purpose of this chapter is to demonstrate that the fears of diagnostic and interventional radiologists can be allayed as long as they keep pace with technological advances in imaging.

## There Is More to the Job of the Radiologist than Looking at Images

The job of the radiologist entails much more than interpreting images in front of a console. The image itself represents only part of the information necessary for correct diagnosis and cannot be dissociated from the patient's clinical and biological history. Oncological decisions are made at multidisciplinary consensus meetings in which the radiologist plays a major role in decision-making and is central to therapeutic reflection by placing image analysis in its overall context. The radiologist also participates in training, teaching, clinical and fundamental research, and the administration of healthcare structures and management—all of which are integral parts of the radiologist's duties. It is difficult to imagine how machines could perform these various functions.

Artificial intelligence tools will help to improve and simulate the organization of diagnostic imaging tests based on a patient's history and symptoms. In this way the indications of imaging examinations, the types of examination to be performed, and automation of the image acquisition protocol can be determined. Once such a review is complete, postprocessing algorithms will increasingly capture more images recording a set of data over protracted periods of time, improving image quality, segmenting the anatomy, and detecting and quantifying biomarkers. For example, much like genomic applications in oncology their "radiomic" counterparts are developing applications making it possible to map different components within the same tumor, which correlates with prognosis of the disease.

Interventional radiology is a separate entity. It finds itself at the crossroads of other medical and surgical specialties, but suffers from the difficulty of recruiting competent specialists. It would greatly benefit from intelligent systems enabling operators to train on mannequins using simulators, guidance, and ballistics to facilitate access to tumor targets. For example, chemotherapy significantly alters the ultrasound visibility of hepatic lesions treated with percutaneous radiofrequency. Innovative software now enables the fusion of scanner images, magnetic resonance imaging (MRI), and positron emission tomography (PET). Their simultaneous display on ultrasound screen makes lesions visible and accessible for percutaneous treatment.

It is difficult to see how a robot could perform endovascular navigation in this way in the near future let alone percutaneous identification and destruction of a liver tumor.

At present diagnostic and interventional radiological reasoning seems to be the hardest thing for artificial intelligence to imitate. It is here that human beings come into their own and play the most important role.

# Who Is Responsible for Medical Liability?

Humans will always have to accept the ultimate responsibility. Aviation is a good model of rigor and perfection that should inspire medicine. In 2017 there were no deaths in commercial flights. This was the result of high-technology automating surveillance and safety tasks normally performed by personnel such as anticollision systems and traffic control. It was also largely due to better training, mandatory training on flight simulation systems, awareness of safety issues, allowing flight crews to report errors without sanction, and listening to their concerns.

In such a model as aviation where automation has made inroads over the past two decades people have more freedom and time to react to an increasing amount of useful information supported by a coherent security awareness environment. However, there has been no decrease in the number of airline pilots—quite the contrary. The comparison between medicine and aviation may appear inappropriate or inaccurate. However, there are characteristics common to both disciplines.

Both focus on the safety of people throughout their travel or care journey. Both rely on human expertise and high-level training to supervise the processes involved. Both have also seen enormous progress in automation in recent decades, and of course both benefit considerably from artificial intelligence systems taking on ever more cognitive and commonplace tasks from humans. However, legal responsibility is the simple reason why humans could not be excluded. It is unimaginable that the inventor of an artificial intelligence system would choose to take full legal responsibility when human lives are at stake. No airline has ever considered flying an unmanned airliner and no insurer would run the risk of endorsing such a proposition.

It is currently the case in medicine for intelligence systems to be used solely as decision aids and to leave final decisions to qualified personnel. No system granted medical regulatory approval has ever claimed to be capable of decision-making unless the decisions made are minor and not life threatening. Indeed, it is impossible for an artificial intelligence system to be 100% accurate at resolving a medical diagnostic issue because medicine remains an art that cannot be fully quantified or resolved. There will always be confounding factors, errors, and reasons that will always need some form of human monitoring. Finally, there is little likelihood of patients in the near future accepting to be cared for and treated entirely by a machine without human intervention when they can be made to feel secure by help provided to doctors by technology.

Intelligent systems that significantly improve the imaging workflow, diagnostic relevance, and dexterity of interventional procedures will lead to greater confidence in and increased demand for medical imaging examinations.

Since the applications of artificial intelligence have become the new standard in imaging it is expected that analysis times will decrease, the risk of reporting errors will be reduced, and there will be a corresponding increase in the demand for imaging and therefore for radiologists.

# What Does the Future Hold for the Radiologist Occupation?

Radiologists in the coming decades will be increasingly freed from routine tasks thanks to prefilled but still verifiable examination reports and user-friendly analysis tools used to release large amounts of radiolabeled data.

Currently, too much time is wasted counting, measuring, and comparing tumors observed on successive scans to see whether chemotherapy is effective knowing full well that the calculation is approximate and does not reflect intrinsic productive transformations within these very tumors. Too much time is wasted counting vertebrae to report the level of metastasis. It is far more preferable to verify that a system has correctly identified all vertebrae and validate its results. Radiologists will go from the status of "ball counters" with coarse tools to that of data controllers processing increasingly sophisticated quantified results.

Moreover, radiologists will be more capable than ever of fulfilling their physician function because of time savings in communicating results to clinicians and patients brought about by artificial intelligence. The profession of radiologist has a reputation for working in the shadows; artificial intelligence has the potential to bring it back into the light.

In conclusion, radiologists have long been aware of artificial intelligence since image reconstruction in the digital age has been based on algorithms. Such algorithms are becoming ever more sophisticated, autonomous, and automatic. This spectacular evolution should be perceived by the radiologist as an aid to diagnosis and image-guided treatment.

We share the conclusions made by Nicholas Ayache at the "Medical imaging and automatic learning: Towards artificial intelligence?" conference when he said, "Artificial intelligence is an ally, through its computerized tools at the service of a more personalized, more precise, more predictive and preventive radiology to better treat the real patient. The master on board will always remain the radiologist with qualities such as compassion, understanding, creativity, critical thinking and professional conscience that artificial intelligence cannot have. Thanks to artificial intelligence and the confidence it will bring to radiological diagnosis and treatment, not only should the number of radiologists increase, but there are other professions to be developed in hospitals such as physicists, programmers, engineers etc. who will work on a daily basis, side by side with radiologists. We must remain vigilant so that those who administer us do not blindly replace people with machines in the field of medical imaging, as has been the case in other sectors."

# Functional Imaging for Customization of Oncology Treatment

Dimitris Visvikis and Catherine Cheze Le Rest

Unlike anatomical imaging the purpose of functional imaging is to highlight the metabolic properties of organs, tissues, or cells—not to identify body structures. Consequently, this type of imaging makes it possible to study pathological processes by the functional and molecular modifications they produce—not by anatomical alterations. Functional imaging by emission tomography has established itself as a major tool in various clinical fields such as oncology, neurology, and cardiology. Positron emission tomography (PET) plays a predominant role in oncology. Diagnosis, the first of the clinical applications, is based primarily on the visual (qualitative) detection of pathological hyperfixation. Such an indication remains unavoidable, but the introduction of multimodal systems coupling a PET detector to a CT scanner (PET/TDM) has helped to develop new indications for PET. The PET/TDM combination makes it possible to have a functional image that is better adjusted than an acquisition made by another machine, at another time, and of another anatomical image and thus to accurately transfer anomalies located on the PET to the anatomical image (Fig. 1). This is the reason functional imaging today also plays an essential role in patient follow-up and therapeutic assessment, as well as in radiotherapy planning.[1] Such new indications are major challenges in the management of patients with the final challenge being personalized treatment. However, the clinical acceptance of multimodality imaging in such new indications clearly implies new developments because it must make it possible to reliably and reproducibly quantify visualized

---

[1] Weber W. A., Figlin R., "Monitoring Cancer Treatment with PET/CT: Does It Make a Difference?" *J Nucl Med*, 2007, 48, 36S–44S; Ford E. C. et al., "FDG PET/CT for image guided and intensity modulated radiotherapy," *J Nucl Med*, 2009, 50, 1655–1665; Jarritt P.H. et al., "The role of PET/CT scanning in radiotherapy treatment planning," *Br J Rad*, 2006, 79, S27–S35.

D. Visvikis (✉) · C. C. Le Rest
INSERM, UMR 1101, University of Brest, LaTIM, Brest 29200, France
e-mail: visvikis.dimitris@univ-brest.fr

C. C. Le Rest
Department of Nuclear Medicine, University of Poitiers, Poitiers, France

© Springer Nature Switzerland AG 2020
B. Nordlinger et al. (eds.), *Healthcare and Artificial Intelligence*,
https://doi.org/10.1007/978-3-030-32161-1_20

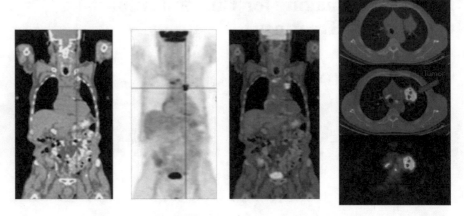

**Fig. 1** 18F-FDG for metabolism imaging with PET/CT. *FDG*, Fluorodeoxyglucose; *PET*, Positron emission tomography; computerised tomography (CT), ???

fixations in terms of activity distribution and tumor volume not only at a given time but also over time (e.g., by following patients during their treatment). Although PET has the advantage of being inherently quantifiable and providing functional information that complements the anatomical information provided by magnetic resonance imaging (MRI) or X-ray computed tomography (CT), its use is made difficult by multiple factors that affect the quality of functional images. These factors include high statistical noise (due to reduced acquisition times[2]), partial volume effects[3] due to the limited spatial resolution of PET (4–5 mm in 3D), and the physiological movements of patients.[4]

Current clinical practice in oncology is still largely based on the visual exploitation of images acquired at different times during patient management (particularly, before treatment, but also during and after treatment for early or final assessment of response to therapy). However, such visual analysis makes quantitative evaluation possible and may limit patient stratification or the possibility of evaluating treatment response. In addition, clues usually extracted manually from the images are subject to high interuser and intrauser variability.

Using activity distribution measurements in functional imaging to characterize tumors may be an advance, but in practice its value is limited because it is most often restricted to measuring maximum intensity within the tumor.[5] This is indeed

[2]Boellaard R. et al., "Effects of noise, image resolution and ROI definition on the accuracy of standard uptake values: A simulation study," *J Nucl Med*, 2004, 45, 1519–1527.

[3]Soret M. et al., "Partial-Volume Effect in PET Tumor Imaging," *J Nucl Med*, 2007, 48, 932–945.

[4]Nehmeh S. et al., "Effect of respiratory gating on quantifying PET images of lung cancer," *J Nucl Med*, 2002, 43, 876–881; Visvikis D. et al., "Respiratory motion correction in PET/CT," *Médecine Nucléaire*, 2007, 31(4), 153–159.

[5]Wahl R. L. et al., "From RECIST to PERCIST: Evolving considerations for PET response criteria in solid tumors," *J Nucl Med*, 2009, 50, 122S–150S.

very reductive because it does not provide any information on the extent of the disease or on the distribution of the tracer within the tumor. It is therefore necessary to develop automatic (or semiautomatic) methodologies capable of defining new indices extracted from PET/CT images to characterize tumors (e.g., by reporting their spatial dimension or local or regional heterogeneity in a precise, robust, and reproducible manner).

## 3D Determination of Tumor Volumes

The first technological block common to all targeted clinical applications is 3D determination of functional volumes.[6] Most of the segmentation methods proposed so far are based on signal strength threshold values in images that are not very robust to noise and contrast variations and unable to manage heterogeneities in the distribution of activity in tumors.[7] The Fuzzy Locally Adaptive Bayesian (FLAB) algorithm is an automatic approach specially adapted to the characteristics of PET images for automatic definition of 3D tumor volumes.[8] To manage the noisy and fuzzy properties of PET images the FLAB algorithm considers each voxel as belonging to a mixture of classes calculating probability depending on the statistical distribution of voxels in the image and their spatial correlation. The statistical measure used combines so-called "hard" Dirac measures with a contiguous "fuzzy" Lebesgue measure to model the presence of homogeneous regions and fuzzy transition zones between these regions.[9] Using the statistical model previously introduced we can only consider binary segmentation such as "object of interest" and "background." If we also want to differentiate between more or less active regions in an object of interest—which will enable us, for example, to modulate the dose delivered to the various components of the tumor target—we need a third hard class such as "background," "low-active tumor," and "high-active tumor." Such a development involves the use of more than two hard classes with fuzzy modeling.[10] We now

---

[6]Jarritt P. H. et al., 2006, art. cit.; Wahl R.L. et al., 2009, art. cit.

[7]Nestle U. et al., "Comparison of Different Methods for Delineation of 18F-FDG PET-Positive Tissue for Target Volume Definition in Radiotherapy of Patients with Non-Small Cell Lung Cancer," *J Nucl Med*, 2005, 46(8), 1342–1348; Daisne J.F. et al., "Tri-dimensional automatic segmentation of PET volumes based on measured source-to-background ratios: Influence of reconstruction algorithms," *Radiotherapy Oncology*, 2003, 69, 247–250; Van Dalen J.A. et al., "A novel iterative method for lesion delineation and volumetric quantification with FDG PET," *Nuclear Medicine Communications*, 2007, 28, 485–493.

[8]Hatt M. et al., "A fuzzy locally adaptive Bayesian segmentation approach for volume determination in PET," *IEEE Trans Med Imag*, 2009, 28(6), 881–893; Hatt M. et al., "Accurate automatic delineation of heterogeneous functional volumes in positron emission tomography for oncology applications," *Int Journal Rad Onc Biol Phys*, 2010, 77, 301–308.

[9]Hatt M. et al., 2009, art. cit.

[10]Hatt M. et al., 2010, art. cit.

consider whether each voxel can belong either to one of the three hard classes or to one of the three fuzzy transitions between one of the three pairs of hard classes.

## New Functional Imaging Indices to Predict Therapeutic Response

Evaluation and temporal monitoring of therapeutic response is one of a number of new applications as a result of evolving multimodal imaging. Beyond evaluation of response there is real interest in identifying factors that predict response, even before treatment begins, to guide and optimize the therapeutic decision. Biological approaches to test ex vivo chemosensitivity from a tumor sample have not yet been successful and do not cover all therapeutic modalities.[11] Functional imaging in such an indication is probably a promising method.[12] Such information as tumor volume, longitudinal extent, or heterogeneity of activity within the tumor are likely to have significant predictive or prognostic value (Fig. 2). Indeed, the level of fixation and spatial distribution of tumor activity are influenced by several underlying physiopathological phenomena that themselves vary within the tumor (hypoxia, metabolism, infusion, proliferation, angiogenesis). Since such conditions at least partly determine response to treatment it is legitimate to believe that the distribution of fixation must be linked to the therapeutic response observed in a given patient.

With this context in mind we have proposed several approaches based on texture analysis.[13] We define texture as a spatial arrangement of a predefined number of voxels allowing the extraction of complex image properties. Such a methodology consists in two steps. First, matrices describing each type of texture on the images are extracted from the previously defined tumor volumes. Then, texture parameters are calculated on these matrices. All the textures considered[14] have been adapted to 3D volumes for this work. Cooccurrence matrices describing voxel–pair arrangements and matrices describing voxel alignments of similar intensity are calculated by considering up to 13 different angular directions. Finally, matrices describing the differences between each voxel and its neighbors and the characteristics of the homogeneous areas of the tumors (number, size, etc.) are calculated. All these parameters

---

[11] Schrag D. et al., "American Society of Clinical Oncology technology assessment: Chemotherapy sensitivity and resistance assays," *J Clin Oncol*, 2004, 22(17), 3631–3638.

[12] Wahl R. L. et al., 2009, art. cit.

[13] Tixier F. et al., "Intra-tumor heterogeneity on baseline 18F-FDG PET images characterized by textural features predicts response to concomitant radio- chemotherapy in esophageal cancer," *J Nucl Med*, 2011, 52, 369–378.

[14] Haralick R.M. et al., "Textural Features for Image Classification," *IEEE Trans Syst Man Cybern*, 1973, 3, 610–621; Loh H. et al., "The analysis of natural textures using run length features," *IEEE Trans. Ind. Electron*, 1988, 35, 323–328; Thibault G. et al., "Texture indexes and gray level size zone matrix: Application to cell nuclei classification," *Pattern Recognition and Information Processing*, 2009, 140–145.

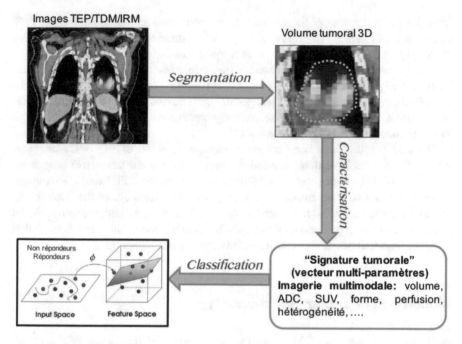

**Fig. 2** Predictive models based on several types of information from multimodal imaging. (ADC: Apparent diffusion coefficient in Magnetic Resonance (MR) diffusion imaging, standardised uptake value (SUV), Computerised tomography (CT), PET (positron emission tomography) *ADC*, ???; *IRM*, ???; *SUV*, ???; *TDM*, ???; *TEP*, ???

are likely to characterize in one way or another the heterogeneity of the tracer in the tumor at various scales (local, regional, or global).

The first clinical study focused on extracting tumor heterogeneity parameters for primary esophageal lesions from pretreatment with fluorodeoxyglucose (18F-FDG) for carbohydrate metabolism imaging of PET images. Such a characterization was compared with the therapeutic response evaluated after treatment according to response evaluation criteria in solid tumors (RECIST) that are based on comparing pretreatment and posttreatment CT anatomical images, the status of complete, partial, or no response having been confirmed by biopsies. The results of this study showed that volume and heterogeneity information extracted in this way from the preprocessing image can predict therapeutic response with high sensitivity and specificity (>80%). On the other hand, simple 18F-FDG accumulation measurements (stabdardised uptake value, SUV) normally used in clinical routine have shown themselves to be of no value in predicting response. A second study of 74 ENT cancer patients retrospectively recruited from two hospitals—Brest (France) and Taoyuan (Taiwan)—reported that heterogeneity ($p < 0.05$) and SUVmax ($p = 0.005$) parameters were independent prognostic factors of TNM stage in the analysis of survival without local recurrence.[15] Such studies have shown that advanced analysis of PET images helps to identify patients at high risk of recurrence and requiring alternative or more intensive treatment and/or more frequent follow-up.

Finally, two recently published studies (including one on a multisite, multicancer cohort of 555 patients) were able to demonstrate the complementary value of different biomarkers (volume and tumor heterogeneity).[16] Thus, in non-small cell lung carcinoma (NSCLC) tumor volume, heterogeneity characterized by entropy, and clinical stage are independent prognostic factors.[17]

To date all studies have been devoted to separate analysis of PET or CT imaging. We are the first to have demonstrated the benefit of a multiparametric prognostic model combining tumor heterogeneity parameters from both PET and CT imaging, functional tumor volume, and clinical stage. This was carried out on the same cohort of NSCLC patients studied in the next section. Indeed, such a multiparametric model has a discriminating power complementary to stratification of the clinical stage that is higher than that of the various biomarkers considered independently.

## Biomarkers of Tumor Heterogeneity

We end this chapter by highlighting the involvement of functional PET imaging and the tumor heterogeneity biomarkers just mentioned in identifying the molecular, genomic, and transcriptomic signature of a tumor thus contributing to the development of increasingly personalized therapeutic orientations. The objective of our study here was to evaluate the relationships between quantitative parameters that can be extracted from 18F-FDG PET images and gene expression profiles obtained by analyzing transcriptomic chips. Our study involved prospectively recruiting 60 patients with ENT cancer and is being conducted at two sites (CHRU Brest and CHU de Poitiers). All patients underwent 18F-FDG PET at diagnosis and were treated with radiochemotherapy. A total of 15 quantitative parameters of tumor heterogeneity could be extracted from PET images. In parallel with the imaging study biopsies were performed on tumors and peripheral healthy tissues for transcriptomic study conducted using Agilent 4 × 44k expression chips. The study identified 1177

---

[15]Tixier F., Hatt M., Cheze-Le Rest C., Ten T.C., Visvikis D., "18F-FDG intra tumor uptake heterogeneity quantification from baseline PET images are prognostic factors of disease free survival and predict local recurrence in head and neck cancer," *J Nucl Med*, 2013, 54, 458.

[16]Hatt M., Majdoub M., Vallières M., Tixier F., Cheze-Le Rest C., Groheux D., Hindié E., Martineau A., Pradier O., Hustinx R., Perdrisot R., Guillevin R., El Naqa I., Visvikis D., "FDG PET uptake characterization through texture analysis: Investigating the complementary nature of heterogeneity and functional tumor volume in a multicancer site patient cohort," *J Nucl Med*, 2015, 56, 38–44; Tixier F., Hatt M., Valla C., Fleury V., Lamour C., Ezzouhri S., Ingrand P., Perdrisot R., Visvikis D., Cheze-Le Rest C., "Visual versus quantitative assessment of intra-tumor 18F-FDG PET uptake heterogeneity: Prognostic value in non-small cell lung cancer," *J Nucl Med*, 2014, 55(8), 1235–1241.

[17]Hatt M., Majdoub M., Vallières M., Tixier F., Cheze-Le Rest C., Groheux D., Hindié E., Martineau A., Pradier O., Hustinx R., Perdrisot R., Guillevin R., El Naqa I., Visvikis D., 2015, art. cit.

genes whose expression varied by a factor of 2 depending on whether healthy or tumor tissue was considered in ENT cancers. Such results were then combined with the imaging data using Genomica module networks. This step made it possible to divide all genes differentially expressed into subgroups of genes coregulated by three parameters from PET imaging. In a final step the functional annotation of these gene subgroups using "Gene Ontology" and the "David" tool made it possible to link PET parameters to annotations and physiological processes. Such processes include the biosynthesis of unsaturated fatty acids (which has already been described in cancer), cell proliferation, signal resistance, apoptosis, and angiogenesis. In conclusion, the quantitative parameters extracted from PET images (particularly, those characterizing tumor heterogeneity) seem to be able to provide information related to underlying physiological processes.[18] However, we clearly need multicenter studies with larger patient cohorts to validate models developed for several types of cancer in monocentric patient groups. At the same time, there seems to be a need to develop methodological approaches for combining heterogeneous information within this type of model to be able to exploit all the parameters that can characterize tumors and their therapeutic response. Finally, artificial intelligence approaches seem essential for the construction of multiparametric models exploiting the plethora of parameters likely to characterize tumors and the large volume of data related to their multicentric nature. In this context, approaches that will allow transfer learning on databases created at each hospital site, without the need to centralize them on single sites, will be preferred to eliminate material constraints, accessibility and data exhaustiveness.

---

[18]Tixier F. et al., "FDG PET derived quantitative heterogeneity features reflect gene expression profiles in head and neck cancer," *J Nucl Med*, 2014, 55, suppl. 1, 450.

# Virtual Image and Pathology

Cécile Badoual

## Introduction

Artificial intelligence (AI) is focusing increasing interest in various domains in our hyperconnected world. In medicine automated machines and diagnostic software are being routinely used by many practitioners (particularly, in biology and radiology). Much like morphologists whose work relies on pattern recognition from pictures, pathologists are particularly affected by the automatization and digitization of techniques. The primary step in everyday lab life is to provide diagnoses from digitized slides with or without computer assistance. A digitized slide corresponds to the scanned image of a colored glass slide. The entire surface of the picture can be explored and any area of interest, just as happens with a traditional microscope, can be zoomed in on. The use of such digitized slides for routine diagnoses is spreading. In the near future they may allow multiparametric approaches to diseases; hence, observation by the trained eyes of pathologists may be combined with computer-assisted pattern recognition, cell counts, or quantification of biomarkers. There is a great deal of hope that such approaches will provide more efficient analysis of complex phenomena such as those implied in cancer.

Moreover, digital pathology is getting easier to use and allows long-distance cooperation. Once confined to educational or research purposes pathological data are shared on social networks with a simplicity that was unthinkable not so long ago. It is now possible to reach colleagues with a few clicks anywhere in the world to establish a diagnosis. What might have taken days or weeks is now becoming incredibly fast.

However, such great progress is accompanied by limitations in the use of digital imagery. First, as happens in a number of areas involving Big Data, information has

C. Badoual (✉)
Department of Pathology, University of Paris Descartes, Paris, France
e-mail: cecile.badoual@aphp.fr

Georges Pompidou European Hospital, APHP, Paris, France

© Springer Nature Switzerland AG 2020
B. Nordlinger et al. (eds.), *Healthcare and Artificial Intelligence*,
https://doi.org/10.1007/978-3-030-32161-1_21

to be protected, labeled, and sorted. Second, improving such information involves the lengthy process of algorithm programming and algorithm teaching. The role played by physicians is crucial to assessing the clinical relevance of such data. This chapter will highlight the need for adaptations and job creation as a result of the revolutionary management of patients and their pathologies brought about by such data.

## Digitized Slides in the Pathologist's Routine: A Revolution

Pathologists by job description establish diagnoses after studying samples at the gross level and then at the microscopic level using thin sections. Analyzing hematoxylin–eosin (HE) stained thin sections represents the main diagnostic activity of pathologists. Complementary techniques may be carried out on request to verify diagnostic hypotheses or to assess prognostic or theranostic criteria. Such hypotheses include immunolabeling with chromogenic or fluorescent revelation in situ hybridization and in some laboratories molecular biology testing. Various clinical, biological, macroscopic, and histological data are integrated to diagnose neoplasia or inflammatory, infectious, or degenerative conditions.

It took less than a decade for slide scanners to appear in the digital pathology field. They quickly gained popularity as their prices became more affordable allowing ever more facilities to be equipped. While white-light or fluorescence microscopes are still routinely used in laboratories, the emergence of such new technologies has revolutionized behavior (Fig. 1). Indeed, there is no need for a microscope when a digitized slide is used. Slides may be accessed either via a shared server or via secure medical networks. Slides may be displayed on remote workstations by several people at the same time, be rapidly sent to colleagues using dedicated servers, and be stored online in the cloud.

We can therefore see that it will only be a matter of time before student teaching, pathologist training, and resident pathologist training will be provided exclusively through this means. Moreover, second-opinion providers, expertise networks, and national or international working groups have become so familiar with digital pathology since it facilitates data sharing and brainstorming of digital slides. Telepathology makes expert meetings easier and less time-consuming now that sharing platforms are replacing multiviewer microscopes. In addition to the use of such platforms in teaching, or expertise digital images, which can be easily annotated, the virtual slides are or will be increasingly present in the routine activity of pathologists. This has prompted some laboratories to make all slides scanned over the years by technicians or secretaries available to allow diagnosis to be carried out only on virtual slides. In addition, since these slides are almost systematically and permanently integrated into the patient's computerized file they are very easily accessible in the event of a recurrence or a request for review. Other facilities have chosen to scan slides representative of cases presented during multidisciplinary meetings enabling better communication with clinicians since factors such as diagnosis and size of excision limits can be discussed while the digitized slide is displayed on screen. Clearly, pathologists will still

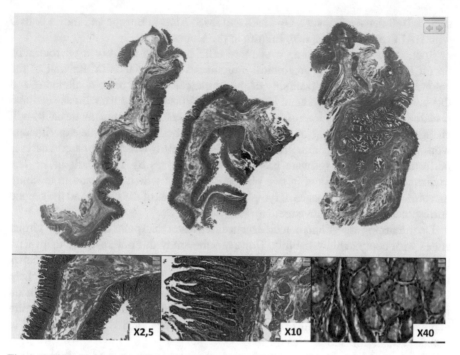

**Fig. 1** Digitized image of a colon sample. Since the virtual slide is not fixed the surface of the slide can be explored and zoomed in on at various magnifications

be needed to read and interpret such slides and pass on their expertise to others. At present senior pathologists find it faster to use microscopes, but younger ones are now well trained in the use of virtual slides. It will take a few more years for the microscope to be abandoned everywhere. This can only happen if the images produced are of perfect quality; can be read on a computer screen, a digital tablet, or even a smartphone; and above all if pathologists sign up to taking the "all digital" path. In light of such data there is an urgent need for careful reflection on their use. Dematerialized slides are personal health data that have to be carefully protected whether they are stored in public or private hospitals. To date no legal text dedicated to this question has provided a sufficiently satisfactory answer in any country. In addition to the data protection issue there is the question of the medical expertise required of pathologists. It is therefore urgent for legislators to define the professional requirements needed for the diagnosis of digitized slides.

However, the most important upcoming revolution will be automated diagnostic decision support for interpretation of digitized slides. It represents the biggest challenge for AI algorithm developers and physicians. For the moment most automated readings are based on the recognition of areas identified a priori by pathologists that can be recognized as a result of learning or teaching. However, an approach without this previous step of manual recognition is also being developed in parallel. There are a number of companies developing analysis software programs across the world such as Definiens©, Tribvn©, Owkin©, and IMSTAR© in Europe and Indica Labs© with HALO and Perkins© with InForm in the United States.

Such software is becoming ever more efficient but is still not used routinely. So far it can differentiate anatomical structures such as glands in the wall of the colon.[1] Recognizing the specificity of the single-cell units is more challenging and this issue will be discussed later. However, the results obtained from cross-sectional research studies are very impressive raising the expectation that diagnostic habits will change with increasing use of "deep learning."[2] A good example is the experimental work carried out by a Dutch group published in *JAMA*, which compared analyses performed by several software programs with analyses by 11 pathologists.[3] The experiment was carried out in two phases the first of which consisted in teaching machines to recognize images of lymph node metastases of the breast and the second corresponded to comparative reading

Deep learning algorithms detected metastases faster than pathologists using virtual slides with comparable reliability. However, the study did not compare them with results obtained by pathologists using microscopes. This preliminary work shows that when it comes to very specific questions software can be of additional help in patient management. Other comparable studies have been carried out both on HE slides and on slides after immunohistochemical or in situ hybridization staining and show encouraging results.[4] Other studies have been carried out such as one in collaboration with Google Health.[5]

Other parameters can be evaluated and explored using these new complementary tools such as automated measurement of the intensity of a staining, quantification of stained cells, automated evaluation of tumor regression grade (TRG) after cancer treatment.[6] The digital analysis of images will eventually make it possible to homogenize certain results and in so doing improve patient care, but this will only be possible if the final results are validated by a pathologist who will be responsible for the diagnosis. Even though interpretations can be automatized, the simple fact is that as a result of the diversity of tissues, cells, stainings, and clinical implications the information still needs to be synthesized and the final diagnosis confirmed.

---

[1] Sirinukunwattana K., Snead D.R.J., Rajpoot N.M., "A stochastic polygons model for glandular structures in colon histology images," *IEEE Trans. Med. Imaging*, 2015, 34, 2366–2378.

[2] Litjens G., Kooi T., Bejnordi B.E., Setio A.A., Ciompi F., Ghafoorian M. et al., "A survey on deep learning in medical image analysis," *Med Image Anal*, December 2017, 42, 60–88.

[3] Bejnordi B.E., Veta M., van Diest P.J., van Ginneken B., Karssemeijer N., Litjens G. et al., "Diagnostic Assessment of Deep Learning Algorithms for Detection of Lymph Node Metastases in Women with Breast Cancer," *JAMA*, 2017, December 12, 318(22), 2199–2210.

[4] Litjens G. et al., art. cit.

[5] Rubbia-Brandt L., Giostra E., Brezault C., Roth A.D., Andres A. et al., "Importance of histological tumor response assessment in predicting the outcome in patients with colorectal liver metastases treated with neo-adjuvant chemotherapy followed by liver surgery," *Ann Oncol*, February 2007, 18(2), 299–304.

[6] Liu Y., Gadepalli K., Norouzi M., Dahl G.E., Kohlberger T., Boyko A., Venugopalan S., Timofeev A., Nelson P.Q., Corrado G.S., Hipp J.D., Peng L., Stumpe M.C., *Detecting Cancer Metastases on Gigapixel Pathology Images*, 2017 arXiv: 1703.02442.

# Multiparametric Approaches: New Opportunity to Refine Our Understanding of Disease

Major progress has been made in patient management in medicine in recent years (particularly, in oncology). Groundbreaking advances in immunotherapy and personalized medicine have allowed improvements in quality of life and survival for many patients. Recently emerged biomarkers are allowing the prediction of treatment response. Many future biomarkers (especially, for the prediction of response to anticancer immunotherapies) are linked to the tumor microenvironment whose analysis has been facilitated by new methodological tools. This is the reason it has become crucial in recent years to develop staining methods and means of interpreting them in the various cellular populations infiltrating or composing a tissue (particularly, in a neoplastic context). To date automated reading techniques have been found to be efficient for simple staining and for immunohistochemical staining[7] under white-light microscopes. Thus, for practical reasons most currently used prognostic immunoscores rely on only one immunohistochemical label per slide. By contrast, single-parameter or multiparameter stainings revealed by fluorescence on a sample section are still most often read and interpreted with the naked eye.[8] The six- to seven-color multiplex labeling technique that takes place on a single paraffin-embedded thin section makes it possible to characterize the different cell types more precisely and to comprehend their functions and interactions within the microenvironment.

Some pathology departments have acquired expertise over the years in using multiple in situ staining methods like these. Until recently it was impossible to automate the acquisition of fluorescent staining for an entire slide so that multiparameter data suitable for research could be acquired (especially, in oncology). Technology now allows automatic acquisition of a large surface or the entire slide within days or even hours with the added advantage of the acquired image being archived. Fast acquisition (milliseconds for each spot lit) is fundamental in fluorescence because it avoids photobleaching (i.e., "bleaching" or "fadding" corresponding to progressive extinction of the fluorescent signal after excitation of the fluorophore during reading under the microscope). This allows the use of multiple and sometimes unstable fluorochromes (such as phycoerythrins), and therefore the use of markers that enable labeling of more than seven different antibodies on the same slide. This is a major technological advance. The technology enabling separate or combined special analysis of more

---

[7] Galon J., Costes A., Sanchez-Cabo F., Kirilovsky A., Mlecnik B., Lagorce-Pagès C., Tosolini M., Camus M., Berger A., Wind P., Zinzindohoué F., Bruneval P., Cugnenc P.H., Trajanoski Z., Fridman W.H., Pagès F., "Type, density, and location of immune cells within human colorectal tumors predict clinical outcome," *Science*, September 29, 2006, 313(5795), 1960–1964.

[8] Salama P., Phillips M., Grieu F., Morris M., Zeps N., Joseph D., Platell C., Iacopetta B., "Tumor-infiltrating FOXP3 + T regulatory cells show strong prognostic significance in colorectal cancer," *J Clin Oncol*, January 10, 2009, 27(2), 186–192.

than seven fluorochromes is unique. For example, the Vectra or Polaris (Perkins) systems allow the capture of information by spectral resolution in the visible and near-infrared bands (bandwidth between 420 and 900 nm). Vectra and Polaris enable extremely precise and fine quantitative management (cell by cell) of the staining of various tissue samples in a light background or in fluorescence. The detection and phenotypic characterization of cells in tissues combined with bioinformatics image analysis is possible using InForm (Perkin Elmer) software.[9]

Autofluorescence reduction technology (ART) is possible using a scanner running InForm. Obviously, the technologies developed for one type of cancer are transposable to other tumor proliferations or inflammatory diseases. The resulting image or digitized slide is a large file stored in a database on a computer server that can be accessed remotely using user-friendly software that reproduces the functions of a microscope. Data archiving therefore becomes digital and not only physical. In addition, such a high-throughput spectral scanner is capable of scanning several dozen slides in a few hours. This is essential when it comes to studying patient cohorts. Finally, digitized slides can be analyzed automatically (cell counting, surface measurements, etc.) using dedicated image analysis software. In particular, such software allows automatic analyses of parameters that would not be accessible for description by the human eye (cell shapes, multiple molecule networks, vascular networks) adding rapidity, precision, and reproducibility to cell counts and staining quantifications (Figs. 2 and 3). Combining different information on the same slide allows the development of new patient management strategies through the identification of "signatures." These new approaches allow cellular interactions to be understood from another viewpoint: it makes it conceivable to find biomarkers in an unsupervised manner without a priori or prior choice highlighting weak or undetected signals that may be called "early warning signals." Despite all the advantages of these new technologies several obstacles still stand in the way of their generalized routine use. First, these technologies run on very sophisticated and expensive machines. Their use must be restricted to experienced users (engineers, researchers, or doctors) involved in bioinformatics. Self-mathematized reading is a real revolution, yet it remains time-consuming and imperfect in terms of data integration. Moreover, training the software remains long and tedious. Finally, the data obtained are massive, hence the name Big Data, and require adequate and secure processing and storage.

---

[9] Badoual C., Hans S., Rodriguez J., Peyrard S., Klein C., Agueznay Nel H., Mosseri V., Laccourreye O., Bruneval P., Fridman W.H., Brasnu D.F., Tartour E., "Prognostic value of tumor-infiltrating CD4 + T-cell subpopulations in head and neck cancers," *Clin Cancer Res*, 2006, 12(2); Granier C., Vinatier E., Colin E., Mandavit M., Dariane C., Verkarre V., Biard L., El Zein R., Lesaffre C., Galy-Fauroux I., Roussel H., De Guillebon E., Blanc C., Saldmann A., Badoual C., Gey A., Tartour É., "Multiplexed Immunofluorescence Analysis and Quantification of Intratumoral PD-1 + Tim-3 + CD8+ T Cells," *J Vis Exp*, February 8, 2018 (132).

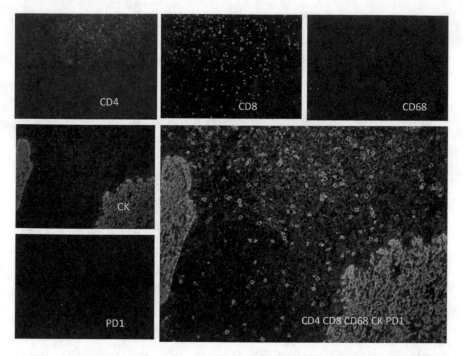

**Fig. 2** Fluorescent multiparametric study of the microenvironment of an ENT cancer: staining of tumor cells with antikeratin (blue), of CD4 T cells (green), of CD8 T cells (pink), of macrophages (purple), of PD1+ cells (red), and of nuclei (blue DAPI)

## Social Networks

Tomorrow's pathologists will be connected to social networks. Evidence for this comes from the United States and Canadian Academy of Pathology (USCAP) whose training and educational courses relative to social networks are aimed toward pathologists of all ages and at all levels of computer knowledge. Facebook with its 2 billion subscribers and Twitter with its 328 million members are the most powerful social networks that can be utilized by medicine (specifically, by pathology).[10] Sharing digitized slides on these platforms is very simple and contributes to learning, to discussing diagnoses, or even to assisting in the diagnostic process (Fig. 4). One or several representative slides can be posted along with comments regarding clinical context, localization of the lesion, etc. Thus, a conversation can start between pathologists from all over the world regarding diagnoses, training, meetings, questionnaires, and hypotheses. Making use of such networks has been shown over time to bring together pathologists interested in the same pathologies.[11]11 Moreover, in

---

[10]Granier C. et al., art. cit.

[11]Isom J., Walsh M., Gardner J.M., "Social Media and Pathology: Where Are We Now and Why Does It Matter?" September 2017, 24(5), 294–303; Gonzalez R.S., Amer S.M., Yahia N.B., Costa

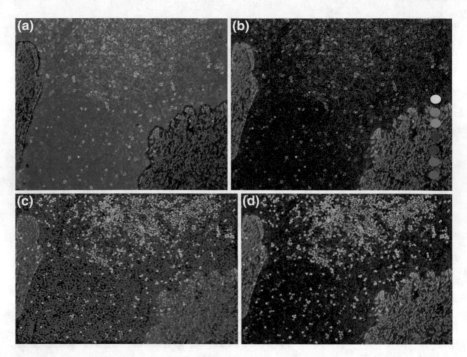

**Fig. 3** Software interpretation of staining in tonsil cancer. **a** Identification and recognition of tumor areas (red) or stroma (green). **b** Identification of differences in staining and color attribution by cell phenotype. **c, d** Research and identification of cells and their phenotypes present on the slide from all the cells of the entire slide or from cells labeled by immunohistochemistry

the work of Jerad Gardner, a young pathologist who is having a meteoric rise to fame in the United States, even legal and ethical impacts have been discussed thanks to social networks.[12] Such questions as data protection and respect for the anonymization of documents produced must be carefully managed so that this health data can be shared by and on behalf of everyone.

## Conclusion and Prospects

Digital pathology has now made it possible to analyze data about tissue images in a more exhaustive way. New Big Data and other data technologies such as deep learning are transforming the profession of the pathologist. Digitized slides and automated analyses will undoubtedly be some of the tools pathologists will use in

F.D., Noatay M. et al., "Facebook Discussion Groups Provide a Robust Worldwide Platform for Free Pathology Education," *Arch Pathol Lab Med*, May 2017, 141(5), 690–695.

[12]Oltulu P., Mannan A.A.S.R., Gardner J.M., "Effective use of Twitter and Facebook in pathology practice," *Hum Pathol*, March 2018, 73, 128–143.

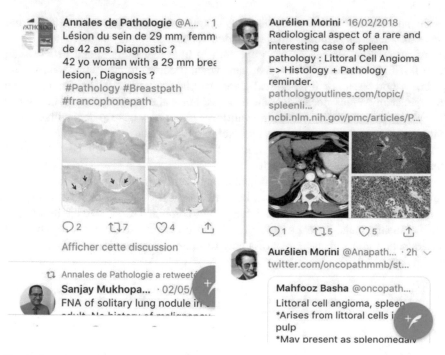

**Fig. 4** Sample messages posted on Twitter by a specialist pathology journal or by pathologists

their daily routine in the near future. When digital pathology becomes part of the daily routine it will likely be restricted initially to simple tasks such as quantifying the immunolabeling of cancer cell nuclei. However, it will not be long after these new technologies are deployed that increasingly complex information will be sought. The technical improvements in research that have emerged in recent years—such as spectral reading scanners, fluorophores adapted to multiparametric in situ analyses, and development of automated counting software—will allow very high–quality multiparametric tissue analysis to be conducted and will become essential for the personalized management of patients and for very detailed study of their pathologies. The development of new techniques will enable, for example, better characterization of cells infiltrating cancers. Such techniques will not only be able to identify on the same slide cell types such as tumor cells and immune cells, but also phenomenal and functional properties such as cytotoxicity, stroma remodeling, ischemic areas, tumor neoangiogenesis, and apoptosis. These new digital imaging techniques are also particularly suitable for the analysis of cellular interactions and the proximity of cells to one another in a given tissue, something that was complicated with conventional immunohistochemistry techniques. Such multiparametric approaches to pathological tissues may uncover crucial information that can rapidly lead to the identification of relevant biomarkers or new therapeutic targets. However, such highly sophisticated techniques are not routinely used.

Social networks will provide an increasingly important space for data sharing since they facilitate sending images needed for teaching and diagnosis and do so in a few minutes. However, it is important to note that using social networks in a professional context requires great care when it comes to ethics and safety. The pathology profession will be radically changed in the context of Big Data and the emergence of "omics" techniques such as genomics and transcriptomics; hence our knowledge of pathologies and their evolution will not only have to deal with clinical data but also radiomics, genomics, and metabolomics data.

Last but not least, this huge mine of information will only be relevant if pathologists learn how to manage it.

Cooperation between medical doctors, engineers, computer scientists, data scientists, and various other actors will be mandatory. The specific skills of everyone involved in this digital transition will have to be combined to achieve the best possible therapeutic management of patients. It is also essential to stress the urgent need for education in the management of a new form of extremely sensitive medical and health data.

# Research

# Artificial Intelligence and Cancer Genomics

**Jean-Philippe Vert**

## Introduction

Cancer affects about 18 million people worldwide each year and is a disease of the genes. Recent advances in genomics are paving the way for the quantitative analysis of large quantities of tumor genomes to better understand the disease and to better orient its treatment by adapting it to the molecular characteristics of each patient. However, to analyze and exploit the flood of genomic data produced everyday ever more powerful algorithms are needed. Artificial intelligence methods such as statistical modeling and machine learning have long played a central role in bioinformatics by automatically capturing patterns and structures in data, classifying and organizing data, and creating predictive models. As we will see in this chapter such approaches are particularly suitable and useful for analyzing data generated by major sequencing programs and addressing many of the challenges of cancer genomics. However, fundamental difficulties will remain until "virtual assistants"—using artificial intelligence to enable effective precision medicine based on the automatic analysis of molecular profiles in clinical practice—appear on the scene.

## Genomics and Cancer

Almost every cell in our body contains our genetic heritage stored in 46 chromosomes. Each chromosome consists of DNA molecules, long polymers that chemically encode a text by successively linking four base bricks called nucleotides and generally represented by the letters A (adenine), C (cytosine), G (guanine), and T (thymine).

J.-P. Vert (✉)
MINES ParisTech, Paris, France
e-mail: Jean-Philippe.Vert@mines-paristech.fr

École Normale Supérieure, Paris, France

© Springer Nature Switzerland AG 2020
B. Nordlinger et al. (eds.), *Healthcare and Artificial Intelligence*,
https://doi.org/10.1007/978-3-030-32161-1_22

In total there are about 6 billion nucleotides that follow one another on about 2 m of deoxyribonucleic acid (DNA) in each cell, which constitutes our genome. This is about 600 times the number of characters in *La recherche du temps perdu*, the world's longest novel according to the *Guinness Book of World Records*. The genome plays a crucial role in each cell since it codes for information that makes possible the synthesis of ribonucleic acids (RNAs) and proteins that are useful for the proper functioning of the cell and the organism. On the other hand, it is the basis for heredity between generations.

Specific to each individual, DNA must be preserved to ensure the proper functioning of each cell in our body. However, alterations in genetic material may occur during life (particularly, during the replication phase of DNA that predistributes each cell division or because of external agents known as mutagens such as ultraviolet rays, tobacco, alcohol, or certain viruses). These are called somatic alterations as opposed to the germline mutations inherited from our parents. Although most of these alterations have no effect on cell function, some may affect important regions of the genome (such as coding for genes or regulatory regions) and result in the inactivation or activation of certain proteins. They can then confer new properties on the cell such as the ability to divide rapidly and prevent cell death. The propagation and accumulation of such alterations during cell divisions can then lead to the emergence of cancer characterized by the rapid and uncontrolled multiplication of cells.

## Clinical Interest

Cancers therefore result from a succession of genetic accidents, and precise knowledge of the alterations involved in a tumor can have multiple clinical interests.

## *Prevention*

Germline mutations are inherited from our parents, are present in all our cells, and can increase our susceptibility to disease. For example, about 2 in 1000 women carry germline mutations in the BRCA1 gene that is involved in DNA repair. These mutations increase the risk for developing breast cancer over a life span by about five times. Indeed, if the molecule encoded by the BRCA1 gene is deficient because of mutation, the number of unrepaired genomic alterations will tend to be high, which constitutes a favorable breeding ground for the accumulation of somatic anomalies and the development of cancer. Knowing our germline genome can therefore help us to have accurate estimates of the risks for developing cancer or other diseases, and to put in place personalized monitoring and prevention strategies. Several commercial companies offer personal genomics services (23andMe, Helix, Veritas Genetics, etc.) that enable everyone to know their genome and their risks for developing various diseases, based on a little saliva and costing a few hundred dollars.

## *Diagnosis*

Somatic alterations specific to cancer cells are acquired over the course of a lifetime. They can be detected by comparing the genome of a cancer cell with that of another supposedly less mutated cell such as blood cells (unless, of course, it is a blood cancer). Early detection of somatic alterations can provide tools for early diagnosis by detecting the appearance of tumors before they are visible in the body.

This is possible, for example, by analyzing the DNA circulating in the blood during routine blood tests because blood in the case of cancer generally contains a small proportion of cancer cells or at least the DNA of these cells. For example, researchers at Johns Hopkins University recently developed a blood test called CancerSEEK to detect 8 common types of cancer including the presence of characteristic mutations in 16 genes in DNA circulating in the blood.[1]

## *Targeted Therapies*

The detection of somatic alterations can also be used to improve and personalize treatment of the disease by using targeted therapies addressing particular molecular abnormalities (e.g., by inhibiting mutated genes in certain tumors; Table 1). There are currently about 50 targeted inhibitors (i.e., drugs on the market) that target a specific gene. Rather than providing treatments based on the type of cancer the trend is to say that a treatment initially targeted for one type of cancer (e.g., breast cancer) could be used for another type of cancer provided the same genomic anomaly is observed. A major step in this direction was taken by the Food and Drug Administration (FDA), which approved in 2017 for the first time the use of a targeted therapy—Keytruda (pembrolizumab)—for any metastatic tumor with a specific genomic anomaly such as deficit in the DNA mismatch repair system (dMMR) regardless of the location of the tumor.

The identification of genetic alterations within cancer cells has led to the identification of new molecular biomarkers. These parameters are now essential for the diagnosis, classification, selection, and monitoring of treatment of an increasing number of cancers. Currently, molecular cancer genetics platforms have a catalog of 60 tests some of which are crucial for access to existing or developing targeted therapies such as the Data Portal of the National Cancer Institute.

---

[1] Cohen J., Li L., Wang Y. et al., "Detection and localization of surgically resectable cancers with a multianalyte blood test," *Science*, 2018, 359, 926–930.

**Table 1** Predictive biomarkers for access to targeted therapy

| Type of cancer | Biomarker | Use of marker |
|---|---|---|
| Breast cancer | Amplification of *HER2* | Prescription of trastuzumab in metastatic breast cancer and adjuvant in early breast cancer |
| | | Prescription of pertuzumab in combination with trastuzumab and docetaxel in metastatic breast cancer |
| | | Prescription of lapatinib in metastatic breast cancer |
| Gastric cancer | Amplification of *HER2* | Prescribing trastuzumab in metastatic gastric cancer |
| Metastatic colorectal cancer | Changes in *KRAS* | Prescription of panitumumab and cetuximab in colorectal cancers without *KRAS* or *NRAS* mutation |
| | Changes in NRAS | |
| | Changes in *BRAFs* | |
| GIST (gastrointestinal stromal tumor) | Transfer of *KIT* | Prescription of imatinib |
| | Transfer from *PDGFRA* | Prescription of imatinib |
| Lung cancer | Mutations of *EGFR* | Prescription of gefitinib, erlotinib, afatinib, or osimeritinib |
| | Translocations of *ALKs* | Prescription of crizotinib or ceritinib |
| | Translocation of ROS1 | Prescription of crizotinib |
| | Changes in *KRAS* | |
| Lung cancer | Changes in *BRAFs* | |
| | Mutations of *PI3KCA* | |
| | Changes in *HER2* | |
| Melanoma | Changes in *BRAFs* | Prescription of vemurafenib, dabrafenib, cobimetinib, or trametinib |
| | *KIT* changes | |
| | Changes in NRAS | |
| Glioblastoma | *MGMT* methylation | Sensitivity with temozolomide |
| Chronic myeloid leukemia (CML)/acute lymphoblastic leukemia (ALL) | Translocation of *BCR-ABL* to diagnosis | Prescription of imatinib or nilotinib as the first line of treatment |
| | Detection of *BCR-ABL* for residual disease monitoring | Imatinib resistance/prescription of dasatinib, bosutinib, or ponatinib as the second or third line of treatment |
| | Transfer of *ABL* | |
| Chronic lymphocytic leukemia | 17p deletion | Prescription of idelalisib |
| | Transfer from *TP53* | |

# Genomic Data

Genomics plays a central role in cancer biology and is increasingly used for the prevention, detection, and treatment of cancers (particularly, with the emergence of targeted therapies). Precision medicine is often used to describe these approaches, which use large amounts of genomic information to develop a patient-specific therapeutic strategy. Let's take a look at where such data come from and how they are processed to finally provide the doctor with therapeutic advice and recommendations.

## DNA Sequencing

It took half a century of scientific discoveries and technological prowess to sequence in the early 2000s the human genome for the first time ever (i.e., to identify the sequence of billions of nucleotides that constitute a genome). Sometimes referred to as the Apollo Biology Project this undertaking paved the way for this immense text to be analyzed. It has provided a better understanding of similarities and differences between species (e.g., that humans and chimpanzees share 98% of their genomes) as well as diversity within a species (e.g., that two human beings share about 99.9% of their genome). Since then technology has progressed at a rapid pace such that sequencing human (or non-human) DNA has almost become a routine operation achievable in a few hours for a few hundred euros.

In parallel other types of sequencing-based technologies have been developed such as analyzing the epigenome (i.e., the set of molecular modifications that act on the function of DNA without altering its code) and studying the transcriptome (i.e., all the small molecules or RNA produced following genome transcription that play a crucial role in protein production and cell function).

Taken together all such data form what can be called the "molecular portrait" of a cell. This molecular portrait makes it possible to differentiate not only individuals, but also cells within an individual. Although all cells in our body have more or less the same DNA, they can have very different molecular portraits (e.g., an expressed neuron will have many RNAs that a skin cell will not express). Drawing a molecular portrait of a tumor cell can also play an important therapeutic part in the diagnosis and treatment of cancer.

## Storing and Handling Millions of Genomes

The use of sequencing data in a clinical setting poses technical problems (particularly, because of the volume of data generated). Depending on what is sequenced (the entire genome or just the coding parts) and what is stored (the raw images produced by the sequencer or just a summary of the sequences found), it takes between 10 gigabytes (GB) and several terabytes (1 TB = 1000 GB) to store the information from a genome on a hard disk. Knowing that cancer affects about 18 million people worldwide each year this would represent at least a few hundred or thousand petabytes (1 PB = 1000 TB) per year should we want to sequence them all. Although such a position has not been reached, massive sequencing plans are being developed around the world. Examples include France Médecine Genomique 2025 whose target is to sequence

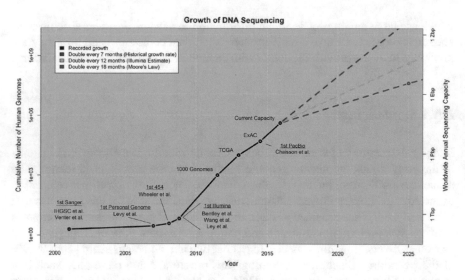

**Fig. 1** Growth in the number of human genomes sequenced. The rapid growth from 2007 to 2008 onward corresponds to the emergence of massive parallel sequencing techniques. By 2025 it is estimated that the number of humans sequenced will be between 100 million and 2 billion. *Source* Stephens ZD, Lee SY, Faghri F, Campbell RH, Zhai C, Efron MJ, et al. (2015) Big Data: Astronomical or Genomical? PLoS Biol 13(7): e1002195. https://doi.org/10.1371/journal.pbio. 1002195

235,000 genomes per year in France, the Obama Precision Medicine Initiative whose target is to sequence a cohort of 1 million volunteers, and China's Precision Medicine Initiative whose target is to sequence about 100 million individuals by 2030. By 2025 it is estimated that the storage of genomic data will require between 2 and 40 exabytes ($1\,EB = 1000\,PB$) (Fig. 1).[2] Although these figures exceed the capacities and expertise of the usual IT infrastructures of hospitals and research centers, they remain comparable with all the videos stored on YouTube. It can therefore be expected that genomic data will increasingly migrate to Big Data professionals as long as they can provide security guarantees compatible with requirements related to the storage of personal data of a medical nature.

## Artificial Intelligence and Genomics

The collection of large amounts of genomic data will pave the way for their exploitation by artificial intelligence methods (in particular, statistical inference and automatic learning) to solve many tasks. Such methods have been at the heart of bioinformatics techniques for the analysis of biological sequences for more than 30 years.

---

[2] According to Stephens Z., Lee S., Faghri F. et al., "Big data: Astronomical of genomical?" *PLoS Biology*, 2015, 13(7), e1002195.

Graphic models and neural networks, for example, have been used since the 1990s to decipher coded information in genomes, infer phylogenies between species, and predict protein structure from their sequences.[3]


## Inferring the Structure of Genomes and the History of Tumors

Artificial intelligence methods enable researchers to get their knowledge included in probabilistic data modeling and then to infer relevant information by letting the algorithm itself optimize model parameters on the real data. In the case of DNA annotation, for example, specific graphic models called hidden Markov chains are used. They make automatic inference of genome annotation (what are the coding regions, promoter regions, etc.) possible from regularities discovered by the model in the DNA sequence. Such methods fall into the category of so-called unsupervised learning methods because they learn to annotate the genome without being provided with explicit information about parts of the genome whose annotation is already known. These graphical models offer great flexibility and can be adapted to various situations. Another more recent application of these methods is to extract epigenetic information (i.e., molecular modifications around DNA). This was done as part of the international ENCODE project in 2012 that was aimed at establishing precise annotation of the functional parts of the human genome based on molecular portraits measured in various cell types.[4] In the context of tumor genomes the graphical models long used to infer phylogenies between species have found an interesting application. From DNA sequenced on a tumor at various times (e.g., at diagnosis and subsequent removal of the tumor) or from samples taken from various parts of the tumor it is possible to characterize heterogeneity within the tumor itself and to reconstruct clonal subpopulations present in the tumor and its evolutionary history in terms of alterations.[5]

Using unsupervised learning tools such as matrix factorization it is even possible to automatically identify the processes involved in tumor onset and progression. For example, it is possible to identify whether a cancer has appeared as a result of exposure to sunlight or tobacco by analyzing mutations observed in the DNA of a tumor.[6] Surprisingly, the matrix-factoring techniques used to carry this out are

---

[3]Durbin R., Eddy S. et al., *Biological Sequence Analysis: Probabilistic Models of Proteins and Nucleic Acids*, Cambridge University Press, 1998; Baldi P., Brunak S., *Bioinformatics: The Machine Learning Approach*, MIT Press, 1998.

[4]Hoffman M., Buske O., Wang J. et al., "Unsupervised pattern discovery in human chromatin structure through genomic segmentation," *Nat Methods*, 2012, 9(5), 473–476.

[5]Brown D., Smeets D., Székely B. et al., "Phylogenetic analysis of metastatic progression in breast cancer using somatic mutations and copy number aberrations," *Nature Communications*, 2017, 8, 14944.

[6]Alexandrov L.B., Nik-Zainal S., Wedge D.C. et al., "Signatures of mutational processes in human cancers," *Nature*, 2013, 500, 415–421.

similar to those used by video-on-demand platforms such as Netflix to customize their recommendations.

## Classifying Tumors

By collecting data on many tumors there is now a means to systematically compare their molecular profiles to identify the presence of recurrent or specific events in one or a subgroup of cancers. Unsupervised dimension reduction or classification techniques can, for example, identify homogeneous subgroups within a heterogeneous population. Such techniques have been used in cancer research since the early 2000s when it became possible to measure the complete transcriptomes of several hundred tumors. Comparing hundreds of molecular portraits in this way revealed the great heterogeneity of certain types of tumors. Breast cancer has been divided into five main classes according to their molecular profiles. This classification is of clinical interest because the prognosis and response to treatment are different for each class (Fig. 2).[7]

## Attending to Therapeutic Choices

In addition to structural inference and unsupervised classification artificial intelligence excels in the art of prediction such as predicting the risk for cancer recurrence and adapting treatment accordingly based on gene expression and mutations in the DNA of a biopsy and predicting the effectiveness of treatment based on the molecular portrait of a cancer. Multiple predictive tasks aimed at providing relevant information for therapeutic decisions are nowadays mainly carried out by supervised statistical learning methods.

Take the example of cancer recurrence risk assessment that can influence the decision to prescribe adjuvant chemotherapy treatments after surgical removal of the tumor. The approach consists in collecting molecular portraits of the tumor from groups of patients at the time of initial diagnosis and then following these patients for several years. A "recurrence" label is associated with molecular portraits of patients in whom a new cancer has appeared in the first five years after initial diagnoses and a "non-recurrence" label is given to others. Then, from such so-called "stretched" data a learning algorithm is developed to predict the tumor category (recurrence or non-recurrence) based on the molecular portrait at the time of the first diagnosis. In practice, genomic data like these are combined with other available information about the disease such as tumor size or patient age that may influence the risk for recurrence.

---

[7]Perou C., Sorlie T., Eisen M.B. et al., "Molecular portraits of human breast tumors," *Nature*, 2000, 406(6797), 747–752.

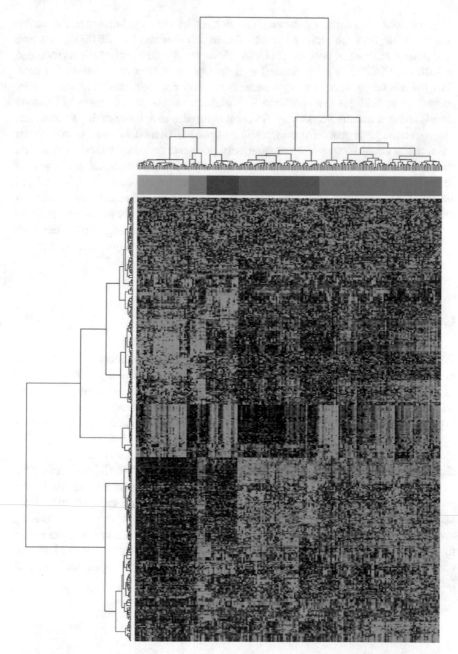

**Fig. 2** Molecular classification of breast cancers. Since the 2000s the analysis of molecular portraits of tumors by transcriptomics (i.e., by measuring the level of expression of 20,000 genes encoded in our genome using technology such as DNA chips) has made it possible to establish a new classification of breast tumors broken down into five subclasses that automatically group tumors expressing the same gene families. In the image each column represents a breast tumor and each line represents a gene. Through the use of sequencing techniques molecular portraits now include not only the transcriptome, but also the genome and epigenome. *DNA*, Deoxyribonucleic acid

Supervised classification is often characterized by the large amount of molecular data available on each patient such as the expression level of 20,000 genes and mutations at millions of positions in DNA. However, the number of patients included in such experiments is often limited to a few hundred or a few thousand at best. This imbalance between the large number of data per individual and the smaller number of individuals is a problematic limitation for the effectiveness of learning algorithms that usually need many different examples to achieve high performance. Moreover, the performance of prognostic and predictive models based on molecular information about tumors remains relatively poor compared with models based on much more summary clinical data. To overcome what statisticians call the "curse of large dimensions" many projects aim to collect data on large cohorts of individuals, as we have seen in this chapter. At the same time, research in mathematics and computer science to improve large-scale statistical learning techniques is in full swing. This is particularly so in combining decades of biomedical knowledge on cancer with automatic learning tools that can analyze the mountains of genomic data we produce every day.

## Conclusion

We are probably at a pivotal time in cancer research. Rapid and concomitant progress in genomics, IT infrastructure, and artificial intelligence over the past two decades has converged into a new way of understanding cancer and its treatment. Many initiatives to collect molecular portraits of large quantities of tumors are under way or in preparation. These coupled with the use of automatic machine learning techniques should improve understanding of the disease at the molecular level and better predict the risks for recurrence and the probabilities of response to various treatments. Such signals will undoubtedly lead to better prevention and more personalized and effective treatment adapted to each patient. Precision medicine will, however, require further progress in our ability to model and analyze genomic data since early attempts from limited numbers of patients did not immediately revolutionize the domain. Promising avenues to overcome these challenges include increasing the number of tumors used to train the models, integrating more biomedical knowledge into these models, and combining genomic data with other types of data such as imaging and medical records.

# Besides the Genome, the Environmentome?

Alain-Jacques Valleron and Pierre Bougnères

The occurrence of disease in humans, their response to treatment, and all their medical history are determined by the products of their genes (gene sequence and gene expression) and of their environmental encounters that do not act independently of each other. Developmental plasticity, epigenetics, and stochasticity govern interactions between environmental factors and gene expression and in so doing make each human phenotype unique. Although considerable (and successful) effort has been made to use all available bioinformatic resources to study the human genome and its individual diversity, the environment has not been subject to the same passion of data scientists.

Huge databases now exist in all areas of the environment and this mass of information will increase exponentially with such developments as the Internet of Things. Such databases can inform the patient's environmentome, which we define as all the environmental data of individuals over the course of their lives. In this chapter we argue that more efforts should be concentrated on this new opportunity to investigate the causality of complex diseases, which ultimately would provide the rationale to include environmental factors in comprehensive precision approach medicine.[1]

The environmentome of a person includes all past exposures to microbes, chemicals, climate, tobacco, and nutrition as well as the history of his/her lifestyle, occupation, stress, and social and economic factors. Although the genome sequence remains unchanged over the course of their lives, humans encounter a myriad of environmental factors from conception to end of life. Such environmental factors modify their immediate physiology and their epigenome in a durable way. It has even been shown

---

[1] National Institutes of Health, *Precision Medicine Initiative: Longer-term Goals*: https://ghr.nlm.nih.gov/primer/precisionmedicine/definition (accessed 2019-05-20).

---

A.-J. Valleron (✉)
Sorbonne University, Paris, France
e-mail: alain-jacques.valleron@inserm.fr

P. Bougnères
University of Paris-Sud, Orsay, France

© Springer Nature Switzerland AG 2020
B. Nordlinger et al. (eds.), *Healthcare and Artificial Intelligence*,
https://doi.org/10.1007/978-3-030-32161-1_23

that the biological memory of events that occurred in parents or grandparents can be transmitted to offspring.[2]

Environmental factors may have an impact on human health by decreasing or increasing their risk for disease. Very few "purely environmental" diseases are known. From one geographical biotope to another or from one society to another the prevalence of major diseases varies due to the exposure of genetically different populations to different environments. It is unlikely that the autoimmune diabetes of a young person from Senegal has the same causes as that of a young person from Finland or Japan. The causality of complex multifactorial diseases is likely to be as heterogeneous as human phenotypes. There is not a single causal path to type 1 or type 2 diabetes, multiple sclerosis, hypertension, or myocardial infarct that would differentiate all cases from all controls.

Let's start with three remarks:

1. The contribution made by genetics to the causality of all major diseases (cancer and cardiovascular, metabolic, respiratory, neurological, and mental disorders, etc.) and of at-risk traits (blood glucose, cholesterol, blood pressure, body mass, etc.) seems to be modest as shown by the following few examples. Comparing genomic variants between cases and controls in 300,000 patients a recent genome-wide association study (GWAS) said that the proportion of blood pressure variance explained by the variability of DNA sequence was only 3.5%.[3] Another observation is the long-known lack of concordance between monozygotic twins who match for type 1 and 2 diabetes only in 23% and 34% of cases.[4] Moreover, a study of 44,766 pairs of twins from northern Europe led to similar conclusions in the field of cancer when both germline and somatic genetic factors are involved.[5] The figures obtained certainly do not accurately measure the situation, but they illustrate the limited share of genetic determinism in the causality of quantitative traits. This makes it clear that non-genetic factors (environment, stochasticity) must fill the gap.

2. Sequencing the human genome in 2000 brought hope and a lot of hype for a short-term revolution in the understanding of major diseases[6] ignoring the illuminating

---

[2]Dias B.G., Ressler K.J., "Parental olfactory experience influences behavior and neural structure in subsequent generations," *Nature Neuroscience* 2014, 17(1), 89.

[3]Ehret G.B., Ferreira T., Chasman D.I., Jackson A.U., Schmidt E.M., Johnson T., Thorleifsson G., Luan J., Donnelly L.A., Kanoni S. et al., "The genetics of blood pressure regulation and its target organs from association studies in 342,415 individuals," *Nat Genet* 2016, 48(10), 1171–1184.

[4]Kaprio J., Tuomilehto J., Koskenvuo M., Romanov K., Reunanen A., Eriksson J., Stengard J., Kesaniemi Y.A., "Concordance for type 1 (insulin-dependent) and type 2 (non-insulin-dependent) diabetes mellitus in a population-based cohort of twins in Finland," *Diabetologia* 1992, 35(11), 1060–1067.

[5]Lichtenstein P., Holm N.V., Verkasalo P.K., Iliadou A., Kaprio J., Koskenvuo M., Pukkala E., Skytthe A., Hemminki K., "Environmental and heritable factors in the causation of cancer analyses of cohorts of twins from Sweden, Denmark, and Finland," *N Engl J Med* 2000, 343(2), 78–85.

[6]Collins F.S., McKusick V.A., "Implications of the Human Genome Project for medical science," *JAMA* 2001, 285(5), 540–544.

remarks and caveats of Lewontin in the early 1970s.[7] It turned out that hundreds of GWASs found a statistically robust association between sequence variants and diseases, but these results saw no revolution in terms of knowledge on the causality of disease nor in the treatment of patients.[8]

3. Until recently efforts devoted to human pathology in terms of biocomputing were focused almost exclusively on genomic data. Each year at the American Medical Informatics Association (AMIA) conference Russ Altman of Stanford University gives a plenary lecture where he comprehensively[9] reviews the previous year's progress in the field of biomedical data analysis regarding genomic, metagenomic, transcriptomic, and epigenomic studies. Surprisingly, progress in the analysis of environmental data is rarely mentioned. Why is the health role played by the environment in humans so constantly advocated, whereas data science studies devote so little space to it?

## The Environmentome: An Object of Analysis Similar to the Genome?

How can the environment be characterized so that it not only improves our understanding of major diseases but also their prevention? It is certainly difficult to imagine that the cause of a disease can be searched for blindly without a precise hypothesis by mixing masses. However, the proof-of-concept of data-driven research has been confirmed by the agnostic approach to hundreds of diseases taken by geneticists. In early studies of complex disease genetics, candidate gene analysis such as human leukocyte antigen (HLA) allowed the low-hanging fruit to be harvested first. GWASs then allowed analyses of the entire genome to test millions of allelic variants (i.e., single-nucleotide polymorphisms or SNPs) on a statistical basis. This has been the case for autoimmune type 1 diabetes ever since HLA class II genes and insulin gene variants were found to be associated in the 1970s. The other 50 predisposing alleles were only identified by comparing tens of thousands of cases and controls for millions of SNPs. Billions of items of data were analyzed to find them. Despite the discovery of diabetes-associated SNPs the genetic causality of type 1 diabetes remains elusive. Since most associated SNPs are not in a coding region of the genome biological explanations have to be sought in regulatory motifs or local epigenomic variation.

When it comes to analyzing the environment the difficulties seem even more formidable. First, although the genome comprises a finite set of billions of nucleotides, the environment in comparison may seem at first glance infinite even though it is not. Second, individual genomic variation is defined by allele genotypes

---

[7]Lewontin R.C., "Annotation: The analysis of variance and the analysis of causes," *Am J Hum Genet* 1974, 26(3), 400–411.

[8]Visscher P.M., Brown M.A., McCarthy M.I., Yang J., "Five years of GWAS discovery," *Am J Hum Genet* 2012, 90(1), 7–24.

[9]Altman R., *Translational Bioinformatics: The Year in Review*: https://rbaltman.wordpress.com/.

(e.g., AA, AT, or TT) that are precise objects of analysis, while the environment cannot be reduced to simple categorical data. Third, part of someone's environmentome prior to contracting a disease is defined by having been at a given place on the planet at and for a given time at a given age. Thus, comparing the whole lifetime environment of cases with that of controls at first sight seems unrealistic. Fourth, traditional environmental epidemiology assesses the association between specific candidate factors and disease in an individual such as cesarean birth, vaccination against measles, the occurrence of chickenpox (which has to be declared in children's health records in France), or the level of tobacco use (personal declaration) simply because such factors in cases and controls are known with acceptable accuracy, whereas environmental epidemiology has a harder time evaluating past exposure to viral infections, pollution, or diet.

The internet era has opened up new horizons for environmental analysis. For example, a woman's pregnancy history and details of her childhood prior to disease onset could reveal important information on the causes of diseases. However, it would certainly be difficult for a woman in her thirties with thyroiditis to start describing her life history from childhood, and obviously impossible for an elderly patient with Alzheimer disease. But, when disease affects relatively young subjects at least some of their life history can be obtained by getting them to fill in a questionnaire—possibly using internet tools—made up of hundreds of random undirected questions (to avoid recall bias): Did your mother have a rash during pregnancy? Was there a dog at home? At what age did you get chickenpox? Did you go to the seaside on vacation? Did you take frequent walks in the forest? Did your parents smoke? Did you eat cereals at breakfast? We have developed such a questionnaire[10] to track salient elements of the family environment before the disease appeared in the patient. Should hundreds or thousands of people answer such a large agnostic questionnaire, this will open up a new avenue in the search for environmental markers of diseases. In combination with the internet such a participatory approach may make this possible in the near future.

Moreover, the environmental exposures children experience are dependent on the geography of their living spaces such as home, outdoors, vacations, school, or travel destinations. Such places are characterized by social factors, proximity to sources of pollution, or climatic characteristics; they also have addresses that can be geolocated and then analyzed by geographical information systems. Since the 1980s geolocations like these have been used to assess specific environmental risks such as air pollution and pesticides. Much more can be done with an agnostic approach where all available geographic information on environmental factors could be used—not just information corresponding to a hypothesis-driven approach.

Let us imagine subject $X$ at time $t$ finding himself at coordinates $(x, y)$ of the planet. The goal is to characterize the various physical, chemical, and social parameters of

---

[10]Balazard F., Le Fur S., Valtat S., Valleron A.J., Bougneres P., Thevenieau D., Coutant R., "Association of environmental markers with childhood type 1 diabetes mellitus revealed by a long questionnaire on early life exposures and lifestyle in a case–control study," *BMC Public Health*, 2016, 16(1), 102.

his environment at each moment of his geographical lifeline. Today, this lifeline is increasingly well known thanks to intrusive geolocation tools that most of us now carry willingly or unknowingly in a smartphone. Once a rich collection of locations is obtained and an "environmental geographical blueprint" can be provided, it is possible to associate the blueprint with numerous environmental databases related to all sectors of the environment. On August 15, 2006 at the age of 8.5 years the subject spent two days in a house located 100 m from a vineyard. For information to be useful environmental databases must have good spatial granularity and be continuously updated. Although current available information is still far from this ideal, there are existing tools that deserve to be considered. Indeed, there already is a myriad of free public environmental data available for extensive exploitation. In addition, specific projects can measure specific personal exposures using sensors and their consequences using toxicological analyses (the "exposome").[11]

## High-Resolution Satellite Databases

An interesting type of huge environmental database collects satellite data providing high-resolution information on land use. The Moderate Resolution Imaging Spectroradiometer (MODIS) created in 1995 uses the Terra and Aqua satellites to capture data and provides a spatial resolution of less than 1 km every other day. The Landsat (USGS–NASA) program began in 1972 and is now in its eighth phase with Landsat 8. Its spatial resolution is 15–60 m and its temporal resolution is 16 days. However, these are the resolutions of the data sources. Processing such data sources to provide usable standard environmental data is time-consuming; hence corresponding databases are not frequently updated because the work of setting up and validating them from the initial raw satellite data is prohibitively long. For example, the Corine Land Cover (CLC) inventory we use shows everywhere in Europe on a 100 m resolution grid and classifies the environment into 44 classes (natural and artificial environments). Thus, the last available CLC database dates back to 2012. In 2010 China launched an ambitious project (GlobeLand30) to provide a 10-class environmental characterization with a granularity of $30 \times 30$ m.[12] Now that the objective of high-resolution geographical description of the surrounding environment has been fulfilled the challenges are, on the one hand, to refine the environmental classifications derived from satellite imagery and, on the other hand, to increase the frequency of publication of corresponding databases. Such issues were the subject of a special volume of the International Society for Photogrammetry and Remote Sensing's (ISPRS) *Journal of*

---

[11]Rappoport S.M., "Implications of the exposome for exposure science," *Journal of Exposure Science and Environmental Epidemiology*, 2011, 21, 5–9.

[12]Chen B., "Global land cover mapping at 30-m resolution: A POK-based operational approach," ISPRS *Journal of Photogrammetry and Remote Sensing* 2015.

*Photogrammetry and Remote Sensing.*[13] Ambitious tools integrating the various data sources (demographic, transport, climate, etc.) using these satellite data are being made available to researchers.[14] The existence of these satellite information systems has already renewed surveillance and alerting for emerging diseases by combining real-time analysis where possible of genomic databases on pathogens with those on the environment. Thus, the analysis of past locations of ebola epidemics in relation to the imaging data collected by MODIS—which finely characterizes altitude, temperature, and evapotranspiration characteristics on a grid $1 \times 1$ km in size—has made it possible to predict sites at risk for harboring the suspected reservoir species (bats) of concern to more than 20 million inhabitants.[15]

We describe below three of our personal attempts using participatory research and environmental databases to search for environment–health associations.

## *Climate Databases to Study the Climate–Environment Relationship*

Health–environment research can be conducted by linking existing environmental and morbidity/mortality databases. For example, the possible impact of a period of extreme temperature during pregnancy on the health of a woman's child could easily be studied by simply correlating existing climate data with the child's health since the latter can be assessed through the National Information System Inter Plans Health Insurance (SNIIRAM).

To study human adaptation to climate change[16] we started from the observation that mortality follows a U-shaped curve as a function of temperature on the day of death or the days preceding death with excess mortality at very cold and very hot temperatures and minimum mortality at intermediate temperatures. With the authorization of the Commission Nationale de l'Informatique et des Libertés (CNIL) we accessed 17 million individual death certificates between 1969 and 2002. The e-obs[17] database provided us with daily variations in meteorological parameters since 1950 within a grid 30 km in size covering the whole of Europe including France. It is therefore possible to study the association between mortality and temperature profiles

---

[13]"Global land cover mapping using Earth observation satellite data: Recent progresses and challenges," ISPRS *Journal of Photogrammetry and Remote Sensing* 2015.

[14]Lloyd C.T., Sorichetta A., Tatem A.J., "High resolution global gridded data for use in population studies," *Sci Data* 2017, 4, 170001.

[15]Haylock M.R., Hofstra N., Klein Tank A.M.G., Klok E.J., Jones P.D., New M., "A European daily high-resolution gridded data set of surface temperature and precipitation for 1950–2006," *Journal of Geophysical Research: Atmospheres*, 2008, 113(D20).

[16]Todd N., Valleron A.J., "Space-Time Covariation of Mortality with Temperature: A Systematic Study of Deaths in France, 1968–2009," *Environ Health Perspect* 2015, 123(7), 659–664.

[17]Haylock M.R., Hofstra N., Klein Tank A.M.G., Klok E.J., Jones P.D., New M., "A European daily high-resolution gridded data set of surface temperature and precipitation for 1950–2006," *Journal of Geophysical Research: Atmospheres*, 2008, 113(D20).

(or other meteorological parameters) on the very day of death or for decades before death. We have shown that when average temperature in France during the summer rises by 1.5 °C there seems to be acclimatization to the warming. Again, without the need for any field data collection and thanks to place of birth being shown on death certificates since 2002 we were also able to show that the relationship between temperature and mortality was similar between a population of immigrants from sub-Saharan Africa and local natives, additional evidence in support to acclimatization.[18]

## *Historical Cohorts to Test Environmental Hypotheses*

One of the major difficulties with environmental epidemiology is that health consequences can be very distant in time from environmental exposures. This can be overcome by using case–control studies, which have sometimes led to great success (particularly, in the fields of cancer and cardiovascular disease). Although the ideal approach would obviously be to study a cohort, it is unfortunately very expensive and takes a long time for results to be provided. Therefore, it is not possible to test environmental assumptions on-the-fly by assembling cohorts. However, there are situations where historical cohorts (i.e., starting in the past) could be constructed by finding past exposures and then correlating them with morbidity and mortality health databases.

To study the long-term health consequences of prenatal stress we used a historical cohort of children whose fathers died in action during the First World War. These children can be identified from birth registers of town halls thanks to the handwritten words "adopted by the nation" written on birth certificates given to wards of the French nation. The use of Big Data enabled us to develop our project. We were able to find fathers who were killed using a database showing 1.3 million deaths in France. The dates of death of war orphans were manually retrieved from death certificates. This showed that children whose fathers' deaths had been announced during the last trimester of intrauterine life—but not before that time nor after birth—had a shorter life span.[19] As causes of death have been shown on death certificates since 1958 it should be possible to compare the causes of death of this cohort with those of the controls. Much of the effort in this work was manual. Students from our team went to town halls to find dusty birth certificates from 1914 to 1916 (>95,000 birth certificates were examined), looked for the handwritten words "adopted by the nation," and then put them in the large army databases identifying the French dead and the French National Institute of Health (INSERM) for the causes of death. Such participatory

---

[18]Mercereau L., Todd N., Rey G., Valleron A.J., "Comparison of the temperature–mortality relationship in foreign born and native born died in France between 2000 and 2009," *Int J Biometeorol* 2017.

[19]Todd N., Valleron A.J., Bougneres P., "Prenatal loss of father during World War One is predictive of a reduced lifespan in adulthood," *Proc Natl Acad Sci USA* 2017, 114(16), 4201–4206.

research involving thousands of volunteers and thousands of town halls with the help of digital tools will make it possible to move to higher levels.

## Case-Only Search for Environmental Causes of Type 1 Diabetes

As a proof-of-concept we studied the environment of a cohort of young people with type 1 diabetes (T1D) (Isis-Diab). One of the constraints we had to face was to work only on cases without controls. Indeed, recruiting "good" controls is a major difficulty and depends on the pathology studied. We wanted to design a method applicable to any disease while knowing only the geographical trajectory of patients prior to disease onset. In fact, disease diagnosis—the only date available to clinicians (unless there is screening)—does not recapitulate disease onset since most diseases have a protracted asymptomatic course where pathogenic mechanisms are already at work. Studying a childhood disease makes it easier to reconstruct this trajectory; hence our choice of T1D. Using a participatory research approach once again, we obtained the address at birth, during pregnancy, and at several ages for the 8000 patients in this cohort. We then linked these locations to geographical databases informing infectious environments. Indeed, since 1984 the Sentinelles network, a real-time computerized system of surveillance of communicable diseases,[20] has been mapping with relatively low geographical resolution the weekly incidence of seven frequently communicable diseases. It was therefore possible to quantify the burden the infectious environment (e.g., chickenpox) placed on children in the cohort during any period between their mothers' pregnancy and their fourth year.[21] By comparing the exposure of patients to various infectious diseases at different ages of their lives with that of "virtual controls" (points randomly drawn from territory proportional to the population density of the same age as the cases), we found that exposure to influenza epidemics and bacterial diarrhea epidemics was positively associated with T1D, whereas a varicella epidemic environment was protective (Fig. 1). Since our patients had been genotyped it was then possible to perform case-only[22] genetic analysis in which environmental exposures are compared with the three genotypes of tens of thousands of SNPs (Fig. 2) and thus come up with hypotheses for gene–environment interaction.

---

[20] Valleron A.J., Bouvet E., Garnerin P., Menares J., Heard I., Letrait S., Lefaucheux J., "A computer network for the surveillance of communicable diseases: The French experiment," *Am J Public Health* 1986, 76(11), 1289–1292.

[21] Bougneres P., Le Fur S., Isis-Diab Collaborative Group, Valtat S., Kamatani Y., Lathrop M., Valleron A.J., "Using spatio-temporal surveillance data to test the infectious environment of children before type 1 diabetes diagnosis," *PLoS One* 2017, 12(2), e0170658.

[22] Khoury M.J., Flanders W.D., "Nontraditional epidemiologic approaches in the analysis of gene–environment interaction: Case–control studies with no controls!" *Am J Epidemiol* 1996, 144(3), 207–213.

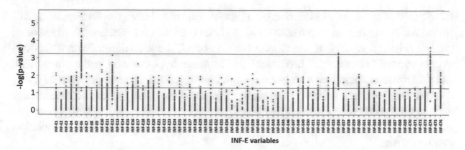

**Fig. 1** Twenty-one signals found in the infectious environment of T1D cases compared with 100 series of "virtual controls". Each abscissa corresponds to children exposed to one of five common infectious diseases at different times (e.g., cumulative exposure to chickenpox epidemics before the age of three years)

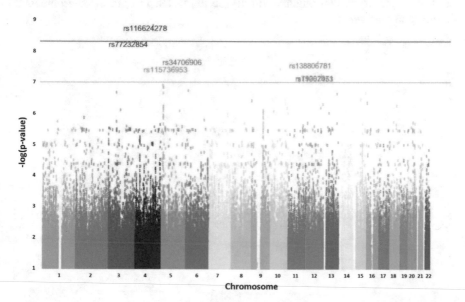

**Fig. 2** Twenty-one pan-genomic analyses of chickenpox exposure before the age of three years (identified as negatively related to the risk of T1D, see Fig. 1)

## Conclusion: Find Environmental Markers First and Then Search for Explanatory Causes

Exploring the environment can lead to apparently strange, yet mysterious results. This is not something to be feared since the identification of predisposing SNPs has not yet led to understanding let alone demonstrating biological phenomena related to SNP genotypes. When we compared the past environment of diabetic children from pregnancy to early childhood with that of controls,[23] using an 845-question all-round questionnaire, in-depth statistical analysis (random forests, propensity scores, etc.) provided a variety of results. On the one hand, the association with infectious events evoked "reasonable" biological and immune hypotheses. On the other hand, the protective association with bee stings, hazelnut cocoa spread, or death of a dog seemed far from any scientific rationality. To the eyes of the scientific community such results seemed less serious than the discovery of an association with a genomic marker. Both, however, deserve the same respect once a robust statistical association can be shown.

This is because markers should not be confused with causes or statistical associations with biological causalities. We must look for environmental tracks to follow with the same passion and energy as geneticists facing the mysteries of genomic associations. We must also be aware that mysteries surrounding the effects of genes on disease predisposition might well only be unraveled in light of environmental factors, and vice versa.

---

[23]Balazard F., Le Fur S., Valtat S., Valleron A.J., Bougneres P., Isis-Diab Collaborative Group, Thevenieau D., Chatel C.F., Desailloud R., Bony-Trifunovic H. et al., "Association of environmental markers with childhood type 1 diabetes mellitus revealed by a long questionnaire on early life exposures and lifestyle in a case-control study," *BMC Public Health* 2016, 16(1), 1021.

# Artificial Intelligence Applied to Oncology

Jean-Yves Blay, Jurgi Camblong and François Sigaux

Western medicine is founded on the notion of medical evidence based on controlled clinical trials and the consensus of expert communities. This practice is robust and responds well to the needs of the so-called "average" patient. However, it lacks the tools and data to implement the recently established notion of precision medicine. Precision medicine in cancerology consists in taking into account the biological characteristics of patients and their tumors, the useful parameters of which are essentially currently provided by genomics and the rapid emergence of expression profiles of both cancer cells and immune cells. To implement such precision medicine practitioners must stay abreast and cope with knowledge of increasing scope and complexity in real time and optimize their analytical processes to take into account the large number of logical rules that quickly arise.

## Challenges of Digital Medicine

### Digital Medicine: Evolution or Revolution?

The idea that machines can help practitioners in the care of patients is not new. Designed as expert systems their algorithms were supposed to mimic the reasoning of specialists in the field. Their principles were essentially based on Bayesian, logical,

J.-Y. Blay (✉)
Léon Bérard Centre, Unicancer, Groupe Sarcome Français, NETSARC, EURACAN, Centre de Recherche en Cancérologie de Lyon, LYRICAN, Université Claude Bernard Lyon 1, Lyon, France
e-mail: jean-yves.blay@lyon.unicancer.fr

J. Camblong
Council for Digital Transformation, Swiss Federal Government, Bern, Switzerland

F. Sigaux
University of Paris Diderot—APHP, Paris, France

© Springer Nature Switzerland AG 2020
B. Nordlinger et al. (eds.), *Healthcare and Artificial Intelligence*,
https://doi.org/10.1007/978-3-030-32161-1_24

or mixed approaches. Although efficient, they have not been able to find a satisfactory place in routine practice within the medical community. The reasons for the failure were due to the lack of real need, the cumbersome means of calculation, and the effort required from practitioners to enter the data since medical records were not computerized.

The current situation is quite different. The needs of precision medicine are considerable. The exponential decrease in the cost of electronic components makes it possible for work to be done on light, connected, powerful, and mobile devices. The internet enables real-time consultations of interconnected knowledge bases. Patient data are increasingly available in digital form, although using the Shared Medical Record in France has not yet been generalized.

Digital medicine can in this sense be considered a means of optimizing personalized access to knowledge and exploiting it in depth. Its area of interest is considerable. However, digital medicine does not represent a revolution in the concepts of diagnosis and therapy, whereas precision medicine is a revolution in terms of approach.

The real revolution in digital medicine will be the ability to use real-life data as a source of knowledge. The data of everyone will thus be at the service of everyone, and the collective experience will be used to build a self-learning system of care.

## Can We Build a Self-learning Health System?

Recording digital representations of individual health data (called digital patients or digital twins) in the same database provides a detailed picture of the diversity of patients at one and the same time. It also makes it possible to analyze the performance of the healthcare system as long as data on the evolution of patients' health status and therapies are entered into the database. Exploitation of such a database by algorithms can help to assist in medical decision-making by identifying the digital family of a given patient. Comparing such changes in patients with their specific management can provide statistical indications to help in decision-making. The data obtained in real life thus complement those obtained by published medical evidence.

In a more ambitious and futuristic vision any elements resulting from analysis of the database can also contribute to the creation of new rules of care that will contribute once validated to medical knowledge thus achieving self-learning in the healthcare system. This vision needs to be monitored in the way it is implemented and used. The quality of the rules will obviously depend on the noise introduced by erroneous data and the degree of information provided by the digital family on which the rule is based. It is also important to note that some rules will be highly dependent on hidden variables inherent in the care system within which these rules have been constructed. They may not be well adapted to another care system.

In any case, using care data in this way could lead to a real revolution in the context of precision medicine with patient experience and physician expertise contributing to greater efficiency and equity.

## Digital Medicine as an Integrating Pillar of the Medicine of the Future

The medicine of the future will be strongly impacted by technological developments already included in the roadmap of many public and private research laboratories. They can be grouped into three strongly linked pillars.

The first pillar is the adoption of multidisciplinary approaches to the development of medical devices for diagnostic, therapeutic, or mixed use. Such devices will benefit from chemistry, synthetic biology, and various fields of physics including electronics and materials science, robotics, and nanotechnologies. Many locks remain to be opened: How can electronic devices that are biocompatible and biodegradable be built? How can nanoobjects capable of imaging and treating lesions be created by interacting à la carte with a particular type of cell (particularly, in cancer)? How can we provide robots with an intelligence capable of anticipating the needs of people with disabilities? Most of these devices through their sensors will contribute to enriching the patient's digital twin in real time.

The second pillar is the biological companion. This includes all personalized biotechnological developments based on elements of the patient's body such as molecules, cells, and tissues. They include the development of organs on chips, the reconstruction of whole vascularized organs, and the genetic modification of immune cells. Personalized cellular immunotherapy approaches in oncology are being developed as is biological reconstruction of tumors ex vivo in 3D form, which is tending to replace transplants in animals poorly describing the complexity of interactions with the immune system in immunocompromised animals. Such reconstructed tumors will make it possible to test the biological hypotheses suggested by systems biology and in silico modeling approaches and thus potentially to evaluate the effectiveness of therapies before administration to the patient.

Finally, the last pillar is the digital pillar integrating the medicine of the future.

The digital doctor–patient relationship can be considered as the frontier between the real world and the virtual world in which three partners interact: knowledge, the digital representation of the patient, and the algorithms (or digital doctor) that interpret the digital patient in the context of knowledge. In such a model the physician can be seen as a mediator whose primary role is to make algorithms and technologies accessible to the patient. Its secondary role—even more essential for the digital doctor–patient relationship—is to understand how the situation of patients in their ordinary life should be adapted to the advice given by algorithms, even if it means sacrificing effectiveness for the optimal well-being of the patient.

## *What Can Be Done to Increase the Chances of Digital Medicine Succeeding?*

Like any major transition the introduction of digital medicine into the healthcare system will be exposed to the hazards of changing a system that brings together patients, healthcare professionals, academic and industrial actors in research and development, and public authorities. Under such circumstances the in-depth analysis of cultural and economic impacts is known to be critical. Although such analysis has not been done so far, a few points can already be outlined.

The training of professionals and keeping the population well informed are two essential points. While digital medical research is inherently multidisciplinary and interdisciplinary, the art of medicine itself will also be transformed. It is already anticipated that the approach to digital medicine by healthcare professionals will require tools to understand the principles of data analysis, system modeling, and decision-making processes. Even though thorough and technical understanding of the algorithms is not necessary, their appropriation is crucial to getting practitioners to adhere to a level of trust that is consistent with their own experience. It is essential not to confine the teaching of mathematics and statistics to the first year of doctor training, but to extend it throughout the initial curriculum. Communicating to the patient what is meant by the digital approach requires finding a means of personalizing the way doctors speak to each patient. Courses in applied psychology could help in adopting such a personalized discourse. Like digital medical research the practice of digital medicine is also inherently multidisciplinary and interdisciplinary; hence new actors such as engineers experienced in multitraining could find a space in the healthcare system.

Digital medicine can be scary because it depends on self-learning about the healthcare system and on altruism from patients entrusting their data to the system. Making the population aware not only of the principles and benefits but also ethical questions of digital medicine will only be really effective if it starts very early in education and probably from middle school. Specific training for teachers in life and earth sciences should be provided. Getting digital media and the public involved in social issues that question ethics committees is a prerequisite to increasing the chances of success.

## Digital Medicine and Artificial Intelligence in Oncology: The Clinician's Vision

The emergence of molecular biology and immunology in the clinical, diagnostic, and therapeutic routine of cancers has led to precision medicine bringing about prolonged survival and sometimes cures in a rapidly increasing number of cancer types. It has also brought about in-depth recomposition of the nosology of such diseases.

The next steps in bringing about this revolution will require integrating artificial intelligence as an aid tool for diagnosis, treatment decisions, and monitoring of treatment by physicians, patients, and caregivers.

## Success of Precision Medicine in Oncology

The nosological classification of human cancers is now based on microscopic morphological analysis often coupled with protein expression in immunohistochemistry and on the measurement of the presence of genomic alterations in cancer cells. The rapid implementation of sequencing panels of genes, exomes, and the entire genome[1]—initially only in fundamental research but then transferred and now made routine in clinics—has made it possible to refine and make nosological classifications more reliable.

These molecular classifications lead to the fragmentation of frequent cancers into a myriad of nosological entities. Routine diagnosis of pilot molecular alterations is now used to guide the implementation of targeted oncogenic treatments and histological classifications of neoplastic maladies of each organ (e.g., adenocarcinoma of the breast or lung). Such diagnoses now need to be supplemented by molecular analyses (HER2, HER1, Alk, Ros, BRAF, Ras, RET, mutations, etc.) to better establish the prognosis and/or guide treatment decisions.[2] Such molecular analyses make it possible to guide the application of specific targeted treatments for these cancers, which could represent 15% of human cancers that present a strong pilot anomaly (i.e., strong driver) making them electively susceptible to a blockage of this signaling pathway.[3]

---

[1] Garraway L.A. Lander E.S. "Lessons from the cancer genome," *Cell*, 2013, 153(1), 17–37; Jensen M.A., Ferretti V., Grossman R.L., Staudt L.M., "The NCI Genomic Data Commons as an engine for precision medicine," *Blood*, July 2017, 130(4), 453–459.

[2] Long G.V., Hauschild A., Santinami M. et al., "Adjuvant Dabrafenib plus Trametinib in Stage III BRAF-Mutated Melanoma," *N Engl J Med.*, 2017, 377, 1813–1823.

[3] Ibid.; Schöffski P., Sufliarsky J., Gelderblom H. et al., "Crizotinib in patients with advanced, inoperable inflammatory myofibroblastic tumors with and without anaplastic lymphoma kinase gene alterations (European Organisation for Research and Treatment of Cancer 90101 CREATE): A multicentre, single-drug, prospective, non-randomised phase 2 trial," *Lancet Respir Med.*, April 2018; Gelderblom H., Cropet C., Chevreau C. et al., "Nilotinib in locally advanced pigmented villonodular synovitis: A multicentre, open-label, single-arm, phase 2 trial," *Lancet Oncol.*, March 2018; Diamond E.L., Subbiah V., Lockhart A.C. et al., "Vemurafenib for BRAF V600-Mutant Erdheim-Chester Disease and Langerhans Cell Histiocytosis: Analysis of Data from the Histology-Independent, Phase 2. Open-label VE-BASKET Study," *JAMA Oncol.*, 2018, 4, 384–388; Casali P.G., Le Cesne A., Poveda et al., "Time to Definitive Failure to the First Tyrosine Kinase Inhibitor in Localized GI Stromal Tumors Treated with Imatinib as an Adjuvant: A European Organisation for Research and Treatment of Cancer Soft Tissue and Bone Sarcoma Group Intergroup Randomized Trial in Collaboration with the Australasian Gastro-Intestinal Trials Group, UNICANCER, French Sarcoma Group, Italian Sarcoma Group, and Spanish Group for Research on Sarcomas," *J Clin Oncol.*, 2015, 33, 4276–4283; Soria J.C., Ohe Y., Vansteenkiste J. et al., "Osimertinib in Untreated EGFR-Mutated Advanced Non-Small-Cell Lung Cancer," *N Engl J Med.*, 2018, 378, 113–125;

In 2010 the Institut national du cancer in France wisely set up a program to characterize molecular anomalies that could be used in this way positioning France at the forefront of nations for molecular epidemiology in the population.[4]

With the significant improvements in survival provided by immunotherapy antiimmune checkpoints (ICPs) on a growing number of cancers—such as non-small cell lung cancer (NSCLC), melanoma, ENT carcinoma, Hodgkin disease, Merkel cell carcinoma, microsatellite instable (MSI) tumors, and mesothelioma—cancer classification now has a new dimension represented by characteristics of the immune stroma: expression of the immune checkpoints (ICPs) PDL1 and PDL2 and the presence and phenotype of infiltrated immune cells such as CD8 T cells, CD4 + Tregs, M2 macrophages, and DC.[5] These characteristics are important predictors of susceptibility to ICP treatments. The mutation load of cancer cells, as well as aneuploidy, are also biomarkers of clinical sensitivity to Ab[6] ICP treatments. Factors predicting the effectiveness of immunotherapy for lung cancer, melanoma, or other cancers are thus multiple, variable according to the cancer, and multidimensional. However, no standardized predictive tools are available in clinical routine to predict the effectiveness of such treatments.

One of the consequences of these developments is the nosological fragmentation of neoplastic diseases. Common cancers then become collections of rare molecular and immunological histological subgroups and are treated individually by various approaches.

However, these approaches describe the neoplastic disease of a given patient from the practitioner's perspective in a complex and still poorly readable way. Apart from the small fraction of cancers where a "strong" pilot molecular alteration has been described, it appears that the majority of cancers result from an accumulation of biological and genetic events heterogeneous in space and time. Their precise

---

Drilon A., Laetsch T.W., Kummar S. et al., "Efficacy of Larotrectinib in TRK Fusion-Positive Cancers in Adults and Children," *N Engl J Med.*, 2018, 378, 731–739; Hyman D.M., Puzanov I., Subbiah V. et al., "Vemurafenib in Multiple Nonmelanoma Cancers with BRAF V600 Mutations," *N Engl J Med.*, 2015, 373, 726–736.

[4]http://www.e-cancer.fr/Professionnels-de-sante/Les-therapies-ciblees/Les-plateformes-de-genetique-moleculaire-des-cancers; Barlesi F., Mazieres J., Merlio J.P. et al., "Biomarkers France contributors. Routine molecular profiling of patients with advanced non-small-cell lung cancer: Results of a 1-year nationwide programme of the French Cooperative Thoracic Intergroup (IFCT)," *Lancet*, 2016, 387(10026), 1415–1426.

[5]Chen D.S., Mellman I., "Elements of cancer immunity and the cancer-immune set point," *Nature*, January 2017, 541(7637), 321–330; Forde P.M., Chaft J.E., Smith K.N. et al., "Neoadjuvant PD-1 Blockade in Resectable Lung Cancer," *N Engl J Med.*, April 2018; Eggermont A.M.M., Blank C.U., Mandala M. et al., "Adjuvant Pembrolizumab versus Placebo in Resected Stage III Melanoma,", *N Engl J Med.*, April 2018; Bellmunt J., de Wit R., Vaughn D.J. et al., "Pembrolizumab as Second-Line Therapy for Advanced Urothelial Carcinoma," *N Engl J Med.*, 2017, 376, 1015–1026; Reck M., Rodríguez-Abreu D., Robinson A.G. et al., "Pembrolizumab versus Chemotherapy for PD-L1-Positive Non-Small-Cell Lung Cancer," *N Engl J Med.*, 2016, 375, 1823–1833; Ferris R.L., Blumenschein G. Jr., Fayette J. et al., "Nivolumab for Recurrent Squamous-Cell Carcinoma of the Head and Neck," *N Engl J Med.*, 2016, 375, 1856–1867; D.T., Uram J.N., Wang H. et al., "PD-1 Blockade in Tumors with Mismatch-Repair Deficiency," *N Engl J Med.*, 2015, 372, 2509–2520.

[6]Chen D.S., Mellman I., 2017, art. cit.

characterization is still unknown to the researcher and the practitioner.[7] Translating this mass of complex information to best serve the patient is therefore an essential task for artificial intelligence in oncology to carry out.

## Integrating Immunological and Constitutional Molecular Complexity to Better Treat Cancers

Digital genetic sequences of genomic alterations of cancer cells are now available in large international databases such as those of the International Cancer Genome Consortium (ICGC) and The Cancer Genome Atlas (TCGA).[8] These databases make it possible to identify new classifications of neoplastic diseases shared by cancers of various histologies and organs. By having similar signaling pathways and multiple signaling pathways various cancers can be activated simultaneously by the same type of cancer. Bioinformatics analyses currently allow new classifications to reclassify diseases. In the future such classifications should guide the application of combined targeted treatments. The same type of approach is used for the immunological classification of cancers, which is at an early stage in distinguishing distinct immunological subgroups shared by cancers of very diverse histologies and organs. Both treatments have issues when it comes to guiding the application of targeted and/or immunological treatments individually and optimizing the development of new targeted or immunotherapeutic treatments in the clinic.

An empirical approach to new immunotherapies and targeted therapies is not possible. The number of molecular subgroups of cancers and the diversity of signaling pathways used and drugs under development require a rational approach to the development of new drugs. The aim here is to make a limited number of clinical trials devoted to ever smaller subgroups of patients feasible. The methodology of clinical trials must evolve to meet challenges that call into question the place of randomization in relation to Bayesian strategies.[9]

[7]Larkin J., Chiarion-Sileni V., Gonzalez R. et al., "Combined Nivolumab and Ipilimumab or Monotherapy in Untreated Melanoma," *N Engl J Med.*, 2015, 373, 23–34.

[8]Blum A., Wang P., Zenklusen J.C., "SnapShot: TCGA-Analyzed Tumors," *Cell*, 2018, 173(2), 530; Liu J., Lichtenberg T., Hoadley K.A. et al., "An Integrated TCGA Pan-Cancer Clinical Data Resource to Drive High- Quality Survival Outcome Analytics," *Cell*, 2018, 173, 400–416.e11; Sanchez- Vega F., Mina M., Armenia J. et al., "Oncogenic Signaling Pathways in The Cancer Genome Atlas," *Cell*, 2018, 173, 321–337.e10; Hoadley K.A., Yau C., Hinoue T. et al., "Cell-of-Origin Patterns Dominate the Molecular Classification of 10,000 Tumors from 33 Types of Cancer," *Cell*, 2018, 173, 291–304.e6; Ding L., Bailey M.H., Porta-Pardo E. et al., "Cancer Genome Atlas Research Network: Perspective on Oncogenic Processes at the End of the Beginning of Cancer Genomics," *Cell*, 2018, 173(2), 305–320.e10.

[9]Saad E.D., Paoletti X., Burzykowski T., Buyse M., "Precision medicine needs randomized clinical trials," *Nat Rev Clin Oncol*, May 2017, 14(5), 317–323; Casali P.G., Bruzzi P., Bogaerts J., Blay J.Y., "Rare Cancers Europe (RCE) Consensus Panel, Rare Cancers Europe (RCE) methodological recommendations for clinical studies in rare cancers: A European consensus position paper," *Ann Oncol*, February 2015, 26(2), 300–306; Buzyn A., Blay J.Y., Hoog-Labouret N. et al., "Equal access

Through the INCa Molecular Platforms Program, France has made molecular characterization platforms available for practitioners to routinely use. This has enabled the molecular epidemiology of several cancer types to be established nationwide. Genomic Medicine 2025 France is a plan that aims to consolidate this position.

Such advances in knowledge have led to the development of innovative therapeutics targeting tumor cells and immunological stromas. Innovative therapeutics have also made it possible to improve patient survival in a new way. We are talking here about precision medicine, a medicine based on science and typified by the rapid evolution of its findings about and effects on increasingly narrow diseases. Oncology is thus at an unprecedented point in the development of knowledge about cancer. This very rapid progression of diagnostic and therapeutic tools raises questions about our ability to establish sustainable therapeutic standards due to the length of time it takes for multiyear changes in therapeutic innovations and the publication of clinical trials to filter through.

## Rare Cancers and Complex Histological Diagnosis

The roles played by experts, pathologists, and molecular biologists in rare cancers have a major impact on the quality of diagnosis, the adherence to clinical practice recommendations, and patient survival. Rare tumors account for 20% of human cancers. However, 30% of cancer deaths are due to delays and inaccuracies in diagnosis. The impact of diagnostic inaccuracies can be demonstrated on survival in a large number of cancers (particularly, in rare tumors such as mesothelioma and sarcoma). It has recently been pointed out that in the absence of centralized pathology review up to 30% of sarcoma diagnoses were inaccurate with significant therapeutic consequences and possible impact on survival.[10] Hence centralized anatomopathological review is necessary and needs to be a part of clinical practice recommendations.

However, such a review is difficult to bring about due to limited expert human resources. In addition, histology, molecular characterization, and immunological phenotyping are often insufficient to accurately diagnose patients even under the best conditions of centralized anatomopathological review. More refined classifications

---

to innovative therapies and precision cancer care," *Nat Rev Clin Oncol*, 2016, 13, 385–393; Casali P.G., Jost L., Sleijfer S., Verweij J., Blay J.Y., ESMO Guidelines Working Group, "Soft tissue sarcomas: ESMO clinical recommendations for diagnosis, treatment and follow-up," *Ann Oncol*, May 2009, 20, suppl. 4, 132–136.

[10]Casali P.G., Jost L., Sleijfer S., Verweij J., Blay J.Y., 2017, art. cit.; Perrier L., Rascle P., Morelle M. et al., "The cost-saving effect of centralized histological reviews with soft tissue and visceral sarcomas, GIST, and desmoid tumors: The experiences of the pathologists of the French Sarcoma Group," *PLoS One*, 2018, 13(4), e0193330.

using new tools are still needed. Artificial intelligence offers such an opportunity to help diagnose rare and complex tumors and explore new dimensions that cannot be seen by the human eye.

This situation can be well illustrated with malignant mesotheliomas (MMs). A recent joint study between Owkin and the Centre Léon Bérard demonstrated the ability of AI tools to help and improve the detection of new nosological entities in tumors.

## Identifying New Predictive Factors in the Effectiveness of Cancer Treatment

The development of new oncology treatments has long followed empirical approaches. The development of targeted oncogenic treatments guided by the presence of an activating mutation (such as the BCR inhibitors ABL, ALK, KIT, HER2, and TRK) has changed this paradigm for a fraction of cancer patients for common cancers such as breast, lung, and colorectal and for rare cancers such as chronic myeloid leukemia (CML) and gastrointestinal stromal tumor (GIST). This fraction continues to grow with new entities identified on a regular basis such as NTRK in 2017. However, even today many targeted treatments such as VEGFR2 or VEGF inhibitors do not have predictive biomarkers. In addition, even the targeted treatments described above have limited and variable efficacy depending on the patient and the predictive tools available, which remain limited.

For immunotherapy with immune checkpoint inhibitors several predictive factors for primary and secondary resistance have been identified such as PDL1 or PDL2 expression (as well as other immune checkpoint (ICP)), mutation load, CD8 infiltrates, aneuploidy, and even intestinal microbiota genotypes. However, biomarkers are numerous; their predictive values are imperfect and vary according to tumor histotypes; and they have not been integrated into a tool that can be used in the clinical routine.

Predictive factors for the efficacy of conventional cytotoxic chemotherapy whether advanced or adjuvant are also poorly characterized. Survival as a result of using these treatments remains limited, although a small fraction of patients benefit from prolonged progression-free and overall survival. Tumor stages, metastasis locations, grade, general tumor status, and age are used to select cytotoxic treatment in advanced stages but are imperfect.

Hinton et al.[11] demonstrated the accuracy and effectiveness of AI tools on visual recognition tasks. Deep-learning methods have been widely used in research making possible the current development of AI applications. The potential applications of these tools are considerable when it comes to analyzing biomedical images from histopathology to radiolabeled or magnetic resonance imaging. These tools make it

---

[11] Krizhevsky A., Sutskever I., Hinton G.E., "Imagenet classification with deep convolutional neural networks," *Advances in Neural Information Processing Systems*, January 2012, 25(2), 1097–1105.

possible for there to be very low error rates for lung cancer classification,[12] cancer detection,[13] and more recently the prediction of mutations from anatomopathological images[14] or the prediction of survival of patient cohorts using a combination of images and molecular data.[15] These initial results demonstrate the potential to develop new tools for diagnosis, prognosis, and prediction of drug response/toxicity in a large number of cancer subtypes using morphology alone, immunohistochemical markers, or combining anatomopathological images with other types of data such as clinical or molecular descriptors. Such tools should facilitate the diagnostic accuracy of pathologists and optimize their work rate. A research program is under way on this topic between Owkin and the Centre Léon Bérard.

## *Integrating Clinical Data from Patient Files*

Computerized records of patients treated for cancer also provide opportunities for the development of algorithms to predict clinical outcomes using AI tools. The potential challenges and obstacles here are numerous such as interoperability of files between institutions, variable richness of reports, lack of standardization of the data to be collected, and data confidentiality.

A major challenge facing AI applied to health data will be integrating simple clinical, biological, radiological, and other data to make the information provided by genomic and immunological histological analyses and algorithms complete. Such information includes the history, associated treatments, and current status of patients. A recent illustration of the need for this approach is the discovery by two large clinical studies that gastrectomy and proton pump inhibitor (PPI) treatment inhibit the antitumor activity of pazopanib, but not other VEGFR2 inhibitors, more than five years after the drug[16] was first marketed.

---

[12]Hou L., Samaras D., Kurc T.M., Gao Y., Davis J.E., Saltz J.H., "Patch- based convolutional neural network for whole slide tissue image classification," *Proceedings of the IEEE Conference on Computer Vision and Pattern Recognition, June–July 2016*, pp. 2424–2433.

[13]Liu Y., Gadepalli K., Norouzi M., Dahl G.E., Kohlberger T., Boyko A., Hipp J. D., "Detecting cancer metastases on gigapixel pathology images," 2017, arXiv Preprint 1703.02442.

[14]Coudray N., Moreira A.L., Sakellaropoulos T., Fenyo D., Razavian N., Tsirigos A., "Classification and Mutation Prediction from Non-Small Cell Lung Cancer Histopathology Images using Deep Learning," 2017, bioRxiv, 197574.

[15]Mobadersany P., Yousefi S., Amgad M., Gutman D.A., Barnholtz- Sloan J.S., Vega J.E.V., Cooper, L.A., "Predicting cancer outcomes from histology and genomics using convolutional networks," *bioRxiv*, 2017, 198010.

[16]Mir O., Cropet C., Toulmonde M., Cesne A.L., Molimard M., Bompas E., Cassier P., Ray-Coquard I., Rios M., Adenis A., Italiano A., Bouché O., Chauzit E., Duffaud F., Bertucci F., Isambert N., Gautier J., Blay J.Y., Pérol D., PAZOGIST Study Group of the French Sarcoma Group– Groupe d'Etude des Tumeurs Osseuses (GSF-GETO), "Pazopanib plus best supportive care versus best supportive care alone in advanced gastrointestinal stromal tumors resistant to imatinib and sunitinib (PAZOGIST): A randomised, multicentre, open-label phase 2 trial," *Lancet Oncol*, May 2016, 17(5), 632–641; Mir O., Touati N., Lia M., Litière S., Le Cesne A., Sleijfer S., Blay J.Y., Leahy M.,

# Artificial Intelligence Applied to Oncology: The Vision of an Industrial Partner

Digital technologies have opened up many opportunities for better diagnosis of diseases and treatment of patients. In particular, next-generation sequencing (NGS) has the potential to provide solutions that should improve the treatment of patients affected by hereditary diseases and cancer. Some 6% of the population are affected by a rare disease[17] and one in two people will be diagnosed with cancer during their lifetime.[18] The analysis of patient DNA and somatic constitution should for all these diseases make it possible to pinpoint the molecular origins of the disease and provide therapeutic approaches that address the cause rather than the consequences (symptoms) of these diseases.

However, digital technologies such as NGS are complex and produce large amounts of data. Protocols for preparing patient DNA samples are not standardized and difficult to standardize because technology and knowledge are constantly evolving and sequencing produces data that contain a lot of bias. This makes it difficult to extract the signal from the noise (detect all genomic variants that are specific to a patient) and to ensure that the same sample from a patient will give the same results in all hospitals.

Algorithmic principles widely used in Big Data activities such as statistical inference, pattern recognition, and automated learning are powerful approaches to ensure post-data production standardization. This approach was adopted by SOPHiA GENETICS and its CEO and cofounder Jurgi Camblong (a visionary entrepreneur pioneering data-driven medicine) and led to the creation of SOPHiA AI. For example, SOPHiA AI makes it possible to reliably detect variations in DNA copies that were not detectable in the past and that can be extremely informative in the case of hereditary diseases such as heart disease.[19] Such a need is even more pronounced for oncology, for tumor heterogeneity, and for the use of chemical agents such as formalin fixed paraffin embedded tissue (FFPE) to fix sections of tumor biopsies making it more difficult to detect somatic mutations specific to a patient's tumor. The detection of mutations from circulating tumor DNA, which has the advantage of avoiding a biopsy and which would allow longitudinal monitoring of the efficacy of

Young R., Mathijssen R.H., Van Erp N.P., Gelderblom A.J., Van der Graaf W.T., Gronchi A., "Impact of concomitant administration of gastric acid suppressive agents and pazopanib on outcomes in soft tissue sarcoma patients treated within the aorta 62043/62072 trials" (submitted).

[17] https://fr.wikipedia.org/wiki/Maladie_rare.

[18] http://www.cancer.ca/fr-ca/about-us/for-media/media-releases/national/2017/canadian-cancer-statistics/?region=qc.

[19] Chanavat V., Janin A., Millat G., "A fast and cost-effective molecular diagnostic tool for genetic diseases involved in sudden cardiac death," *Clin Chim Acta*, January 2016, 453, 80–85; Chauveau S., Janin A., Till M., Morel E., Chevalier P., Millat G., "Early repolarization syndrome caused by de novo duplication of KCND3 detected by next-generation sequencing," *Heart Rhythm Case Rep*, 2017, 3, 574–578.

a therapeutic approach,[20] is routinely performed for the detection of point mutations of the EGFR gene in lung cancer, but is not accessible at this stage to larger and more complex analyses such as whole-exome sequencing (WES).

As President Barack Obama said at the launch of the Cancer Moonshot Initiative in 2016 the development of digital technologies such as the NGS and its combination with artificial intelligence offers hope for turning cancer into a chronic disease. This will require the creation of hospital networks pooling molecular information on patients' cancers and sharing their experience on treatments that have worked or failed in these same patients to create a collective intelligence at the service of all hospitals and patients who would benefit from such networks. This is the task that SOPHiA GENETICS has been working on since 2011 and that had already caught the attention of the European Commission in a report on innovation in Europe to President Jean-Claude Juncker.[21] The same strategy is implemented in the FMG2025 program.

These initiatives require strict data protection control[22] to ensure that they are used exclusively for the benefit of patients and not to restrict their rights or options. Europe with its General Regulation on Data Protection, which has been in force since May 2018, has the means to create a secure environment to ensure the necessary trust for the deployment of platforms that will drive the networks of medical experts. By deploying its secure platform, through which hospitals can gain access to SOPHiA AI, more than 430 university hospitals and cancer centers in 60 countries use SOPHiA AI daily to make medical decisions. By adding broader information on histology and stage treatments that patients have received and the effectiveness of these treatments such a tool as SOPHiA AI offers the potential to position patient cancers in virtual clusters. This paves the way for the use of AI to guide the treatment of an individual patient by drawing on the accumulated experience of thousands of others sharing common clinical and molecular characteristics.

Such AI-based medicine involves sharing and pooling the most effective data and tools provided by all stakeholders. At a time when the population is aging and the sources of social security systems are reaching the limits of their financial capacity, it is essential to have decision support tools that make it possible to target the right treatment even more precisely at the right time. Although this is a major challenge,

---

[20]Bettegowda C., Sausen M., Leary R.J., Kinde I., Wang Y., Agrawal N., Bartlett B.R., Wang H., Luber B., Alani R.M., Antonarakis E.S., Azad N.S., Bardelli A., Brem H., Cameron J.L., Lee C.C., Fecher L.A., Gallia G.L., Gibbs P., Le D., Giuntoli R.L., Goggins M., Hogarty M.D., Holdhoff M., Hong S.M., Jiao Y., Juhl H.H., Kim J.J., Siravegna G., Laheru D.A., Lauricella C., Lim M., Lipson E.J., Marie S.K., Netto G.J., Oliner K.S., Olivi A., Olsson L., Riggins G.J., Sartore-Bianchi A., Schmidt K., Shih L.M., Oba- Shinjo S.M., Siena S., Theodorescu D., Tie J., Harkins T.T., Veronese S., Wang T.L., Weingart J.D., Wolfgang C.L., Wood L.D., Xing D., Hruban R.H., Wu J., Allen P.J., Schmidt C.M., Choti M.A., Velculescu V.E., Kinzler K.W., Vogelstein B., Papadopoulos N., Diaz LA Jr., "Detection of circulating tumor DNA in early- and late-stage human malignancies," *Sci Transl Med*, 201, 6(224), 224ra24.

[21]https://obamawhitehouse.archives.gov/the-press-office/2016/10/17/remarks-president-and-vice-president-cancer-moonshot-report.

[22]https://www.sophiagenetics.com/fileadmin/documents/pdf/Article/Opportunity_now.pdf.

it is one that aims to offer the most democratic approach possible to all patients in a territory composed of urban and rural regions such as France and Europe.

## Conclusion

The applications of AI in oncology clinics are thus multiple from the part it plays in diagnostic assistance, to identification of new nosological entities, to individual treatment guidance, and to the development of new drugs. Such applications will only be feasible if tools capable of ensuring database interoperability are used and wholesale changes are made in the way computerized patient records are recorded.

The real revolution in digital medicine will be the ability to use real-life data as a source of knowledge. The data of everyone will thus be at the service of everyone, and the collective experience will be used to build a self-learning system of care.

# Physical and Mathematical Modeling in Oncology: Examples

Martine Ben Amar

Transdisciplinary research in oncology is constantly being promoted in all the scientific policies of research institutions from scientific programs to calls for tenders. Theoretical methods aimed at better understanding oncology or at improving detection and care techniques are in full development attracting ever younger researchers, mathematicians, or physicists. These methods require biological experiments conducted as part of single-cell recordings, or of many cells. But they will also benefit from temporal acquisitions which should be available in the age of Big Data. However, cancer is a disease of the body and access to clinical data is essential to determining problems to be investigated and to helping get a better understanding of this disease. For many Big Data and cancer is first and foremost the genome and its multiple mutations within tumors. In this chapter we will discuss various aspects that have been or will be the subject of important theoretical developments not only involving new concepts but also including fundamental disciplines. Then we will focus on solid tumors—their shapes, growth, and environment—to give precise examples of what can be achieved through dialogue between Big Data, health data, models, and concepts.

## Current Main Lines of Theoretical Oncology

The phenotypic and genetic heterogeneity of cancer cell populations within the same tumor is increasingly invoked with good reason to explain unexpected failures of therapies targeting a specific signaling pathway or the expression of a particular gene. This heterogeneity concerns such factors as proliferation, apoptosis, differentiation, and resistance to treatment. Heterogeneity must be measured over a large number

M. Ben Amar (✉)
Laboratory of Physics, École Normale Supérieure, Paris, France
e-mail: benamar@lps.ens.fr

Institute of Cancerology of Sorbonne University, Paris, France

© Springer Nature Switzerland AG 2020
B. Nordlinger et al. (eds.), *Healthcare and Artificial Intelligence*,
https://doi.org/10.1007/978-3-030-32161-1_25

of cells and with a resolution in time that goes beyond the simple before and after. Indeed, we must not forget the adaptability of cancer cell populations to a changing environment (i.e., their plasticity), which is one of the main causes of therapy failure. To obtain optimized temporal patterns of drug delivery—even personalized drug delivery—adaptive therapy must take into account this cancer-specific characteristic.

The tumor microenvironment plays a key role in the proliferation of cancer cells (e.g., adipocytes and fibroblasts transformed in breast cancer[1]). Such a microenvironment deserves to be studied and targeted as much as possible by complementary cancer treatments in its two aspects: the influence of the stroma on the tumor and that of the tumor on the stroma. This can only be done by further measuring and recording the changing elastic properties of the stroma. In the case of desmoplastic tumors (of the pancreas, for example) a fibrous collagen barrier surrounds the tumor making it untreatable. However, it is strange to think that we know the genome of very many living species but that we know almost nothing about the elasticity of our tissues with the exception of the heart and arteries. We know almost nothing about the dynamical behavior and mechanics of our tissues over long periods of time, which are essential data for tumor growth.

The immune system as a whole—not just its active mechanism (i.e., the cellular and humoral immune response in cancer)—certainly takes into account control of the fixed parts of the genome related to the self, but also probably control of the variable parts related to the various cellular phenotypes. This field of research is evolving rapidly as a result of intense activity by biologists and oncologists. It should be noted, however, that it remains largely misunderstood. What really happens between cancer cells and those of the immune system, innate or adaptive, when the latter are capable of colonizing or disintegrating spheroids in vitro? It would be very useful if researchers could make available, through databases, the spatial compositions and distributions of T cells in real tumors that are commonly detected by biopsy. This would make it possible to understand, for example, the role of drug treatments sometimes found empirically and could open up new avenues for understanding not only remarkable recent successes, but also a number of unexplained failures of immunotherapy for cancers.[2]

Resistance to cancer treatments brought on by the drugs themselves demonstrates the capability of cancer cell populations to adapt. Such resistance is the subject of numerous theoretical studies and frequent biological observations. Such work most often focuses on resistance mechanisms such as enzymes for intracellular detoxification or DNA repair. However, it is only recently that epigenetic mechanisms have been implicated in completely reversible resistance. Similarly, "bet hedging," a term used in ecology and finance, refers to the strategy of risk minimization consisting in "not putting all your eggs in one basket." In the case of a population of cancer cells

---

[1] Dirat B., Bochet L., Dabek M., Daviaud D., Dauvillier S., Majed B., Wang Y.Y., Meulle, A., Salles B., Le Gonidec S. et al., "Cancer-associated adipocytes exhibit an activated phenotype and contribute to breast cancer invasion," *Cancer Research*, 2011, 71(7), 2455–2465.

[2] Sharma P., Allison J.P., "Immune Checkpoint Targeting in Cancer Therapy: Toward Combination Strategies with Curative Potential," *Cell*, 2015, 161, 205–214.

facing extreme stress, such as exposure to a massive dose of a cytotoxic molecule, bet hedging is an appropriate term to explain the various mechanisms responding to this stress. Optimizing cancer treatment in the clinic is still largely empirical, although this issue has generated theoretical work in optimization and optimal control aimed either at minimizing toxic side effects on healthy cell populations or avoiding the prevalence of resistant cells, but rarely both. This is changing.

When considering such aspects and their relation to cancer biology, improvements in traditional detection techniques brought about by physicists should not be overlooked. They are an integral part of hospital or city services. Improving image analysis (i.e., information that can be extracted from radiographs) is crucial for earlier detection of malignancy. This is a field in which computer scientists and mathematicians are very active. Wavelet theory is one of these techniques. Yves Meyer played a pivotal role in its development and was recently awarded the Abel Prize. An example is given below.

This is not an exhaustive list of cancer-related topics that physicists and mathematicians can be expected to deal with more effectively as ever more information on cancer becomes accessible. Major themes likely developed in the next decade cannot of course be taken into consideration. However, to illustrate what can be expected from modeling at the dawn of Big Data, we will present two examples concerning tumor heterogeneity and microenvironment that will benefit the development of imaging, although this particular field remains a real challenge for information storage.

## Development of Solid Tumors

Solid tumors originate in epithelial tissues that often delimit the walls of organs. These are sites of cell proliferation where cells need to be renewed by a balance between birth and death. In the case of cancer, this balance is unfortunately broken. A mass appears that will compete with other cells and elements of the organ for space and nutrients triggering mechanical forces that in turn will trigger biochemical signals. These will modify cancer cells and their environment. Clearly, it will be difficult to explain the shape (even macroscopically) of the tumor radiologists are trying to determine to help surgeons. Yet physicists and mathematicians know how much the dynamics of forms tells us about the more microscopic processes they are trying to understand. In the case of cancer, these processes aim only at invading the organ and ultimately the organism. The immune system will be the first to react using weapons that are complex and not fully understood at the moment. The next line of defense will be clinicians through surgery, radiology, and medication.

Understanding life and its various forms is a real challenge for physicists and mathematicians irrespective of whether we are dealing with plants, algae, fungi, or animals. Such a challenge started a very long time ago probably by the Greeks. More recently the challenge was taken up by biologists such as D'Arcy Thompson[3] or mathematicians such as Alan Turing[4] both of whom helped to lay the mathematical foundations of the growing living world. In addition to the interactions and forces involved, which remain to be defined, the global form does not result simply from simple addition of individual processes and requires a formalism that is not only technically difficult at the mathematical level, but does not allow us to include the entire state of our knowledge. The task of modern researchers is to make approximations and get to the essentials. However, these approximations will have to be controlled and validated by software developed to deal with mathematical problems by researchers. At all levels from knowledge of phenomena, evaluation of their importance over time, to mathematical modeling we will need data on living organisms to quantify, eliminate, sort, or even validate the importance of microscopic iterations not only in their natural development but also in the presence of disturbances. Apart from agents of the immune system these also include drug agents and radiological or thermal treatments.

There are in vitro laboratory experiments where cancer cells are positioned within a limited perimeter and form a proliferating aggregate called a spheroid, which can then be subjected to such disrupters. Such highly controlled experiments are valuable because they enable us to vary relevant parameters in a controlled way and teach us a lot about cell–cell or chemical signal–cell interactions. However, they will never represent the complexity of the tumor in the organ, the ability of tumor cells to diversify and transform to adapt, and their ability to divert the immune system, for example, to make it complicit in the metastatic phase. Cancer modeling even when limited to solid tumor cases is clearly very complex. However, such modeling above all lacks data on which to base advanced concepts. Such data could be provided by health databases that will likely appear in the next decade.

Biophysical models combined with mathematics and numerical algorithms have made it possible to explain and quantify the evolution of cancer from primary tumor to metastasis development. Such models essentially use partial differential equations (PDEs) or agent-based models that become PDEs by averaging individual cellular behaviors. They are perfectly adapted to representation and prediction of the transient or stationary behavior of cancerous populations. They are good candidates to use to represent a heterogeneous tumor in interaction with its stroma and are well suited to optimize treatment. It is possible to add specific properties called traits to account for biological variability. Metabolism (nutrients, glucose, oxygen) is easily introduced via simplified reaction–diffusion equations where temporal dynamics is often ignored.

An example is given in Fig. 1 where "numerical" melanomas are represented in parallel with melanomas observed in dermatology. As they develop they have a very irregular outline and pigment spots that are explained by the energy between cells varying according to the local concentration of cancer cells. They are few in number at first, the nevus is round and homogeneously brown, and can be confused with moles.

---

[3]Thompson W.D., *On Growth and Form*, Cambridge University Press, 1917.

[4]Turing A.M., "The chemical basis of morphogenesis," *Philos. Trans. R. Soc. London*, Ser. B, 1952.

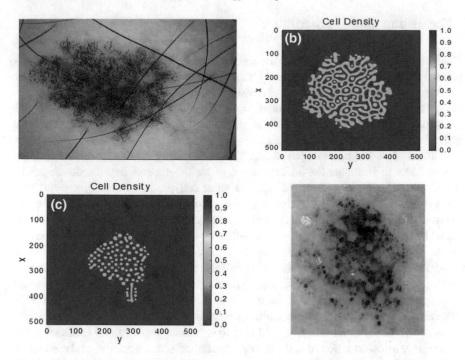

Fig. 1 Characteristic morphology of melanomas (Balois T., Ben Amar M., art. cit.; Xu J. et al, "Analysis of globule types in malignant melanoma," *Arch Dermatol*, 2009, 145(11), 1245.). Note the irregular shape of the tumor and the inhomogeneous color reflecting the inhomogeneous concentration of cancerous melanocytes in the middle of healthy keratinocytes. **b** and **c** Numerical simulations of a model with two types of cells, healthy and cancerous, that separate as the tumor grows resulting in an inhomogeneous concentration. Two types of patterns are possible in numerical simulations and observed in skin tumors: distorted labyrinths or points called nests. They are part of a dermatologist's diagnosis

However, the appearance of spots (part of the alarm criteria for dermatologists[5]) reflects the physical property of separation of cellular aggregates called spinodal transition by physicists[6] and "nests" by clinicians. It is not specific to melanoma and is found in different types of cancers and in in vitro cultures. However, the advantage of skin tumors to modeling is their accessibility because dermatology is very well documented. Such models could shed light on the role played by immune system cells and provide a better understanding of immunotherapies. Laboratory experiments to form cancerous aggregates in the presence of these cells, coupled with modeling, would provide us with information on the dynamics of exchanges between them that changes over time, as mentioned above.

---

[5]Chatelain C., Ben Amar M., "Morphogenesis of early stage melanoma," *EPJ P*, 2015, 130, 8176.

[6]Balois T., Ben Amar M., "Morphology of melanocytic lesions in situ,", *Nature*, 2014, Scientific Reports 4, 3622.

# The Tumor and Its Stroma

The past 30 years have witnessed the emergence of concepts such as microenvironments and stem cell niches not only as regulators of tissue specificity and tumor control, but also in the initiation and development (metastasis) of cancer.[7] The ongoing dialogue between stem cells and their microenvironment (their niche) is essential to regulating their asymmetric division and their future. On the one hand, the niche helps to maintain a set of quiescent stem cells and when necessary facilitates their proliferation to respond to a physiological demand or injury. On the other hand, the niche helps to stimulate the differentiation of stem cells enabling the development of organs. During asymmetric division a stem cell produces a daughter cell that retains its stem character and another daughter cell that can differentiate to adapt to surrounding tissues. Any imbalance between activation and differentiation can "damage" them and make them "cancerous" either by overpopulating the microcolony of stem cells or by aborting their speciation. Under homeostatic conditions (i.e., non-pathological) the niche stroma including cellular and extracellular elements (such as collagen fibers, fibronectin, and laminin) participates in the biochemical and biomechanical control of cancer stem cells to maintain tissue integrity and architecture. This explains why many tumors can remain dormant or progress very slowly. Destabilization of this tissue homeostasis would lead to a "tumorigenic" niche facilitating the oncogenic transformation of cells, their proliferation, tissue invasion, and metastatic escape. This symbiosis of stromal and tumor cells deserves to be studied bilaterally (considering not only cancer cells but also those of their microenvironment). Understanding how cancer cells interact dynamically with stromal cells will open up new avenues of research, define more global cancer diagnosis methods, and extend treatment protocols to all cellular and tissue actors for better patient management (better dosed, individualized, and better tolerated treatments).

Mathematicians and physicists already have the tools and systemic models to enable them to probe the dialogue between cancerous and stromal cells. The dynamics of physiological signals and their alteration by cancer are key to future advances in oncology. We will now describe an investigation method based on signals detected by infrared (IR) thermal cameras and analyzed by wavelet theory. Of course, other techniques are under development such as shear wave ultrasound and computed tomography (CT) scans.

This type of approach can be exemplified by revisiting the use of infrared (IR) thermography for breast cancer diagnosis as a dynamic IR diagnostic tool. Indeed, since the presence of a tumor leads to an abnormal increase in metabolic activity and vascularization of surrounding tissue, IR thermography has long been considered a promising non-invasive screening method for breast cancer. However, it quickly encountered problems such as the lack of sensitivity of sensors to detect deep lesions and a lack of understanding the spatiotemporal processes of thermal regulation of living tissues. The advent of dynamic IR imaging, thanks to the development of

---

[7]Bissell M.J., Hines W.C., "Why don't we get more cancer? A proposed role of the microenvironment in restraining cancer progression," *Nat. Med.*, 2011, 17, 320–329.

digital IR thermal cameras with high cadence (70 Hz) and high sensitivity (0.08 °C), combined with a better understanding of tumor angiogenesis has given new impetus to this field of research. In a recent study the use of time–frequency signal analysis based on the 1D[8] wavelet transform revealed that skin temperature signals showed significant changes around malignant breast tumors. These signals lose their original complexity due to the disorganization of breast tissue.

Comparing thermographic images with multiresolution analysis of mammography of the same patients using 2D wavelet transformation (a kind of mathematical microscope), has recently shown the strong concordance and complementarity of these two techniques[9] (Fig. 2). Should it be shown that such a drastic simplification of thermal signals results from an increase in blood flow and cellular activity associated with the presence of a tumor, it is also certainly the signature of certain architectural changes in the tumor's microenvironment, as X-ray imaging seems to confirm. These results hold great promise for screening techniques currently used in hospitals to detect physiological and architectural alterations that indicate a deregulation of malignant cells and their environment. They will undoubtedly open up new avenues for the implementation of computer-assisted methods (analysis of patient follow-up, longitudinal studies) to assist in the early diagnosis of breast cancer. This approach could be generalized to "surface" cancers such as skin or connective tissue cancers. The development of thermal-imaging probes would be an interesting way to combine them with acoustic and optical probes that are already operational.

## Conclusion

Oncology will benefit from the development of computer techniques at all levels from data analysis and collection, image analysis and storage, to time tracking.

Since current models are often based on instantaneous knowledge and do not always allow access to the way in which cells and tissues transform in the presence of malignant cells within the organism, it is difficult to understand developments (especially, in the presence of treatments). This chapter does not claim to be exhaustive since other avenues based on the theories of evolution are under way.

This chapter is the result of discussions and exchanges with Alain Arnéodo, Jean Clairambaut, and Jacques Prost all of whom I would like to thank most sincerely.

---

[8] Arneodo A., Audit B., Kestener P., Roux S.G., "Wavelet-based multifractal analysis," *Scholarpedia*, 2008, 3, 4103.

[9] Gerasimova-Chechkina E., Toner B., Marin Z., Audit B., Roux S.G., Argoul F., Khalil A., Gileva O., Argoul F., Naimark O., Arneodo A., "Comparative multifractal analysis of dynamic infrared thermograms and X-ray mammograms enlightens changes in the environment of malignant tumors," *Front. Physiol.*, 2016, 7, 336.

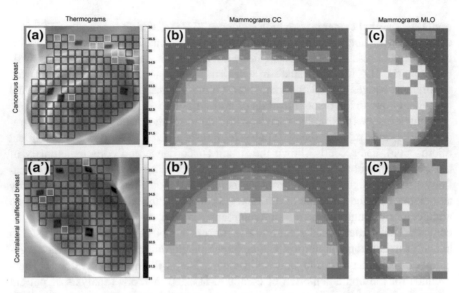

**Fig. 2** Segmentation of suspicious regions based on wavelet (multifractal) analysis of dynamic IR thermograms and mammograms (X-rays). The patient selected for this illustration has a straight cancerous breast (**A–C**) and an unaffected left breast (**A′–C′**). **A, A′** Multifractal analysis (transformed into 1D wavelets) of temporal fluctuations of the skin temperature recorded for 10 min with a high-resolution IR camera in which squares covering $10 \times 10$ mm$^2$ ($8 \times 8$ pixel$^2$) were coded according to the monofractal (*red*) or multifractal (*blue*) nature of temperature–time fluctuations. **B, B′** Multifractal analysis (transformed into 2D wavelets) of the spatial roughness of mammograms for the CC mammographic view in which squares covering $12.8 \times 12.8$ mm$^2$ ($256 \times 256$ pixels$^2$) were coded according to the presence of anticorrelations (*blue*), long-range correlations (*red*), or no correlations (*yellow*). **C, C′** Same as (**B, B′**) for the CC mammographic view. We can see that the regions identified as suspicious—namely, the *red* squares on the thermograms (**A, A′**) and the *yellow* squares on the mammograms (**B, C, B′, C′**)—are concentrated on the left breast in the region where a tumor was identified by biopsy and finally extracted (Ibid). *CC*, Craniocaudal; *MLO*, mediolateral oblique

# Artificial Intelligence for Medical and Pharmaceutical Research: Can Artificial Intelligence Help in the Discovery and Development of New Drugs?

Gilles Wainrib

**Abstract** The digitalization of biology and medicine is producing an exponential amount of data. Combined with the emergence of new analytical AI tools, unprecedented opportunities to accelerate medical progress are emerging. Today, two major areas are about to undergo a profound transformation: medical and pharmaceutical research as well as clinical practice from diagnosis to therapeutic management. Can AI help in the discovery and development of better drugs?

Artificial intelligence (AI) has grown considerably in recent years. AI is far from new supported as it is by a long history that can be traced back to the middle of the 20th century (i.e., to the very moment computers were invented). Indeed, the invention of the computer was based on simplifying calculation, a type of AI. Very early on two schools of thought relating to AI were formed. The symbolists sought to recreate the intellect by positioning themselves at the level of abstraction of logic based on architectures separating memory from computing power as is the case with current computers. The connexionists believed in the possibility of emulating intelligence by imitating the way in which the brain and its billions of interconnected neurons function biologically subtly mixing memory and calculation and offering potentially phenomenal learning capacity. Despite initial enthusiasm and renewed interest in the 1990s following invention of the gradient backpropagation algorithm these connexionist approaches have never really succeeded in breaking through (particularly, on the major classic problems of AI such as image recognition, speech recognition, and machine translation) because they actually require access to huge amounts of data and very high computing power.

It was not until 2012 when the founding article[1] was published that researchers succeeded in making these deep-learning systems work on the problem of image recognition. This was done by combining access to a large annotated database, clever

---

[1] Krizhevsky A., Sutskever I., Hinton G.E., "Imagenet classification with deep convolutional neural networks," *Advances in Neural Information Processing Systems*, 2012, 1097–1105.

---

G. Wainrib (✉)
Owkin Inc., New York, USA
e-mail: gilles.wainrib@owkin.com

© Springer Nature Switzerland AG 2020
B. Nordlinger et al. (eds.), *Healthcare and Artificial Intelligence*,
https://doi.org/10.1007/978-3-030-32161-1_26

use of graphic processing units initially intended for the visual rendering of video games, and subtle mastery of certain algorithmic details. What is now called AI essentially covers somewhat abusively these machine-learning techniques. The enthusiasm was immediate because the improvement in performance was astounding. The article was followed by many studies showing the ability of such an algorithm to solve other tasks related to sound analysis and text analysis that were previously treated by very different algorithmic approaches. Deep learning recently enabled the scientific and engineering community to find a unified biomimetic algorithmic framework that allows unprecedentedly powerful analysis of very complex perceptual signals such as images, time signals, and language. This incredible leap forward opened up new application possibilities in almost every industrial field to such an extent that one of the pioneers of these technologies Andrew Ng called AI "the new electricity."

The health sector is one of these applications and is currently concentrating such enthusiasm that it is becoming the priority of IT giants. Indeed, the digitalization of biology and medicine and in so doing producing an exponential amount of data combined with the emergence of new analytical AI tools offer unprecedented opportunities to accelerate medical progress. Today, two major areas are about to undergo a profound transformation: medical and pharmaceutical research as well as clinical practice from diagnosis to therapeutic management. Although much work (particularly, in medical image analysis) has paved the way for AI to be integrated as a tool to assist doctors in diagnostic or therapeutic decision-making, it is against a background of the fantasies this can generate and all the inertia of health systems that the authors of this chapter decided to focus on the first field—research and development (R&D)—because they believed this field can actually benefit much more quickly from the contributions of AI and have a potential revolutionary impact.

Can artificial intelligence help in the discovery and development of new drugs?

## Fundamental Research

Before discussing drug design or development it is important to consider how applications of AI are affecting basic research in biology and medicine. Put simply, machine learning techniques are increasingly being used to complement statistics by integrating unstructured data such as images, signals, and texts in addition to the structured data traditionally processed by statistics and by capturing complex and non-linear interactions between variables whose number is growing much faster than the number of samples.

When the fundamental role statistics plays is known it will be possible to imagine the impact such methodological advances can have on the biomedical research process.

Although serendipity[2] has led to several major discoveries, the key to finding new treatments is most often a better understanding of the disease. Such an understanding usually begins with a simple question: What are the differences between healthy and sick individuals? This is done by making a number of measurements or observations on healthy and diseased populations of individuals from the clinical level to the microscopic level, seeking to discover disease characteristics, and extracting an understanding of its root causes and the mechanisms that explain the disease. Looking at this problem from the perspective of machine learning it can simply be identified as a classification problem: Can a learning algorithm be taught to distinguish between a healthy man and a sick man? Could this be done with the aim of analyzing how the algorithm would make such a classification and *ultimately* discover new therapeutic targets—not with the aim of making it an automatic diagnostic system? This approach is termed "supervised learning–reverse engineering of the algorithm." Although this approach is far from easy and has many technical challenges such as interpretability and bias, it can also be applied to predicting disease progression to discover the factors explaining why some patients have a more or less aggressive version of the disease. For example, it is now possible to analyze large quantities of histopathology images digitized at very high resolution (several billion pixels) with different immunohistochemical markings and ask deep-learning algorithms to predict the survival time of patients with a given type of cancer by combining these incredibly rich images[3]. In several recent studies such an approach has produced prognostic models based solely on raw images that achieve state-of-the-art predictive performance. In addition to images such approaches make it possible to effectively combine images with biological variables such as genetic mutations or gene expression measures in an integrative way.[4]

In addition to classifying patients as ill vs. healthy making it possible to understand the causes of the onset of the disease and predicting disease evolution making it possible to better understand heterogeneity among patients these approaches can also be used to predict the effects of treatments both in terms of response and toxicity. Since the effects of drugs are very often heterogeneous the supervised learning problem then becomes: How to predict right responders from wrong responders or how to predict patients who will experience severe toxicity? Again, AI techniques enable predictive models to be trained to answer these questions provided that a sufficient number of examples properly annotated are available. Although immunotherapy approaches today offer great hope for the treatment of many cancers, it is still very difficult to understand why some patients have a good response to treatment while others do not

---

[2]Serendipity is the act of making a scientific discovery or technological invention unexpectedly as a result of a combination of chance circumstances and very often in the context of research on another subject.

[3]Courtiol, P., Maussion, C., Moarii, M. et al. Deep learning-based classification of mesothelioma improves prediction of patient outcome. Nat Med 25, 1519–1525 (2019). https://doi.org/10.1038/s41591-019-0583-3

[4]Mobadersany P., Yousefi S., Amgad M., Gutman D.A., Barnholtz-Sloan J.S., Vega J.E.V., Cooper L.A., "Predicting cancer outcomes from histology and genomics using convolutional networks," *Proceedings of the National Academy of Sciences*, 2018, 201717139.

respond or have serious autoimmune responses. Integrating all microscopic images of tumors, radiology, molecular markers, and patient clinical information using such machine learning approaches could lead to better understanding why these treatments do not work on a large proportion of patients. This would have a number of consequences such as improving management by better orienting prescriptions, discovering how to improve existing treatments, and inventing the next generation of immunotherapies.

The discussion in the remainder of this section turns to considering the applications of machine learning technologies in pharmaceutical R&D. However, it is important to remember at this stage that although such deep-learning technologies have been the prominent feature of the last five years, they still have a number of limitations. Two limitations often talked about are the need to feed such algorithms with gigantic quantities of annotated data, and their black box character that prevents explanation of how trained algorithms work. While both these limitations are real, researchers have made significant progress in the use of transfer learning and interpretability techniques to address them. Two other aspects are less often mentioned. First, all machine learning methods share a number of problems with statistics in general. In particular, the study of medical data often faces the two major problems of heterogeneity and bias. These two problems require real reflection when applying machine learning techniques because otherwise the models thus learned may make no sense and may not be very generalized outside the learning domain, even though they may show good performance in cross-validation. Second, convolutional neural networks supporting deep learning are very well adapted to signal data such as image, sound, time series, sequence, and text because such signals have an internal structure with very strong invariant properties despite being classified as unstructured data. When attempting to apply deep-learning methods to traditional tabular structured data it becomes apparent that such methods do not provide any improvement over regularized linear or tree-based methods such as random forests or boosting gradients. Deep learning therefore brings value today to everything dealing with the study of unstructured signal-type data. It is important to be aware of this when striving to enhance innovation in the pharmaceutical R&D process. Although machine learning can generally also be applied to structured data and still bring value, these are older techniques that have already been applied for some time in many industries including chemistry. This neatly leads on directly to this chapter's second section on pharmaceutical R&D process.

## Pharmaceutical Research and Development

Pharmaceutical R&D can be divided into the two main areas of drug discovery and drug development in the context of clinical trials. In this section these two areas will be examined in a very partial way on the basis of some examples of processes that could greatly benefit from new AI technologies.

Drug discovery is a very complex, time-consuming, and costly process that requires teams and resources of the highest technical level. Whether through rational approaches based on target identification followed by iterative molecule design to improve affinity, non-toxicity, and ADME[5] properties, or through more systematic high-throughput screening approaches, they are research processes that generate very large amounts of data.

For several decades now chemists have wanted to use the power of computers to simulate and predict the properties of chemical molecules. One goal is to be able to predict the affinity of a molecule with a therapeutic target of interest or with a target to avoid. If such predictions could be made with great precision, then it would be possible to imagine exploring in silico the space of molecules and finding by calculation what today takes years of intensive research.

The two approaches that coexist here are the physical approach to modeling based on simulating the laws of physics at the atomic level, and the statistical approach that uses learning models to predict the properties of molecules from a large number of experimentally measured examples. Both approaches have their advantages and disadvantages in terms of robustness and computing speed, but they are still far from achieving the dream of the "magic bullet" that would generate the perfect molecule for a target of interest. This is the reason many academic and industrial researchers including a number of startups such as Atomwise are seeking to develop approaches based on deep learning in the hope of bringing the same revolution to this field as happened with image and speech analysis. However, deep learning about this type of data has not to date provided superior performance compared with the application of older learning methods combined with the expert feature engineering. The two main obstacles concern algorithms that must be adapted to the graphical nature of chemical objects and their 3D structure, and access to large databases of high-quality experimental measurements that are now highly confidential and well protected by industry. By combining innovative approaches to graph convolution with federated learning that respect the confidentiality of multiple databases it is hoped that a new generation of molecular activity prediction systems will emerge in the coming years that will have a major impact on the drug discovery process. Moreover, the Innovative Medicine Initiative (IMI) has clearly understood the challenges now that ten European pharmaceutical companies are now collaborating in the MELLODDY project for the development of a federated learning project that respects the confidentiality of partners' data to give themselves the opportunity to be the first to master the revolutionary potential of this technology[6]. However, the path may well still be long and delicate, and other very different approaches such as quantum computation may prove to be more effective and faster than expected.

In addition to resolving computational chemistry issues deep-learning technologies also promise significant benefits in high-throughput analysis (particularly, those based on the analysis of images of cell lines subjected to a combination of different compounds). Such high-content screening approaches generate large quantities of

---

[5] Absorption, distribution, metabolism, excretion.

[6] https://www.ft.com/content/ef7be832-86d0-11e9-a028-86cea8523dc2

images. Research labs and some startups such as Recursion Pharmaceuticals are currently developing ambitious research programs to apply AI to this type of data with the aim of automating systematic screening approaches in an unprecedented way.

The drug development process is based on the conduct of a series of clinical trials and is likely to benefit greatly from AI and the new data analysis and predictive modeling capabilities AI provides.

The last part of this chapter covers three areas that are beginning to be impacted by AI: patient recruitment in trials, the problem of objectivity in the measurement of clinical markers (endpoints) in studies, and the stratification of clinical trials.

Patient recruitment for clinical trials is a very difficult subject. Inefficiencies in matching patients to clinical trials are problematic not only for institutions (be they industrial, hospital, or academic) involved in the development of new treatments, but also for patients themselves who may be missing out on clinical trials that could help them (especially, when it comes to serious diseases where there is a scarcity of effective treatments on the market). The simple objective is to automatically find all patients who could benefit from a clinical trial from a list of inclusion and exclusion criteria or, vice versa, to suggest for a given patient all clinical trials in which they could be admitted. Now that medical records are computerized this task not only seems affordable, but it is thought it would also be appropriate to search hospital medical records by criteria to find eligible patients. However, this type of research is hampered by the complexity of inclusion/exclusion criteria and by the fact that clinical databases are only very partially structured. Most of the information necessary to assess a patient's eligibility for a trial is actually contained in medical reports. Even if the problem of their dispersal was resolved, it is not immediately possible to automatically verify eligibility from such reports. Automatic natural language analysis is one of the areas that is developing rapidly today thanks to advances in deep learning making it possible to consider intelligent systems for patient–clinical trial matching in the coming years.

Patient recruitment for clinical trials is not the only area that can be improved by AI. At the other end of the chain there is trial validation based on evaluating a clinical marker of interest. In oncology, for example, it may be imaging markers that evaluate the decrease in tumor size or the number of tumor lesions. In such a case evaluation of these criteria must be done in a very precise manner because this can have a significant impact on decisions about whether to market new treatments. However, there is generally high variability between observers (here radiologists) who do not always agree on the assessment. Automatic image analysis could standardize this type of evaluation and make it more accurate and reproducible thus allowing the effectiveness of treatments tested in clinical trials to be assessed as effectively as possible.

Although patient recruitment and objectification of measurement are important elements in improving drug development, the subject that probably opens the most exciting perspectives is that of intelligent patient stratification for the various phases of trials. Many trials fail because the criteria defining the indication and target population are not optimal. After years of research to find a good molecule and numerous tests to evaluate its safety the challenge is to understand the heterogeneity of responses and to be able to predetermine and identify the largest possible group of patients who will benefit most from therapeutic innovation compared with a placebo or with reference treatments. AI technologies make it possible today to deepen this type of analysis of treatment–response prediction and predictive biomarker research by integrating ever-more multimodal data including raw data such as anatomopathic images or ECG signals. Since these data cannot be analyzed by conventional statistical analysis tools they have often been overlooked to the extent that still today even in the largest pharmaceutical companies it is difficult to collect all these multimodal data to assess the relevance of machine learning approaches. However, the movement has begun and most stakeholders are moving toward integrating these tools to optimize drug development because the benefits can be decisive in such a competitive industrial environment. Many challenges remain in this field of AI applications. A prominent challenge that needs to be highlighted is the issue of small datasets. Indeed, clinical trials rarely include more than a few hundred patients; hence it may be difficult to operate AI tools with so few learning samples in the same way that statistics are implemented in the problem of multiple tests. To overcome this, transfer-based learning approaches enable algorithms to be pretrained on large datasets (e.g., accessible real-life data) and to complete the training on the smallest datasets in clinical trials. It is therefore by moving toward greater integration of clinical trial data with real-life data that the full power of AI can be brought to bear on drug development and by further aligning the strengths of pharmaceutical companies' R&D portfolios with the most relevant stratifications to provide patients with the most differentiated treatments.

# Open Science and Open Data: Accelerating Scientific Research

Mehdi Benchoufi and Olivier de Fresnoye

> *Knowledge is the only material that grows by sharing it.*
> —Plato

According to Wikipedia "open data"[1] are data freely available for everyone to use and republish as they wish without restrictions from copyright, patents, or other mechanisms of control. Public information is therefore considered "a common good"[2] whose dissemination is of public and general interest.

Wikipedia defines "open science"[3] as a movement making scientific research (including publications, data, physical samples, and software) and its dissemination accessible to all levels of an inquiring society, amateur or professional.

Open data are to open science what the staff is to the musical note. They are its support structure, the conditions necessary for its understanding, its dynamics, and dare we say its key. To ensure the potential of open science is deployed so that there is an inclusive scientific praxis enriched by free contributions, it is essential that the data, information, methods, and results are fully accessible by all and for all. To ensure that the conditions are met, it is necessary to build a legal, operational, and principled framework that takes into account the anonymization of data when they are personal in nature to ensure that contributions are properly respected.

The fundamentals underlying the production of science have long lacked rigidity and links with academic institutions used to be much looser than those of today. Consider Evariste Galois who wrote major articles on the history of science despite not having attended any university. Consider Rousseau reading *Le Mercure de France*

---

[1] https://fr.wikipedia.org/wiki/Open_data.
[2] https://fr.wikipedia.org/wiki/Bien_communal.
[3] https://fr.wikipedia.org/wiki/Science_open.

---

M. Benchoufi · O. de Fresnoye (✉)
Faculty of Medicine, University of Paris Descartes, INSERM UMR1153, Centre d'Épidémiologie Clinique, Hôpital Hôtel Dieu, HP Paris, France
e-mail: olivierdefresnoye@gmail.com

© Springer Nature Switzerland AG 2020
B. Nordlinger et al. (eds.), *Healthcare and Artificial Intelligence*,
https://doi.org/10.1007/978-3-030-32161-1_27

215

whose attention was caught by a message from the Académie de Dijon calling for an essay on a subject formulated as: "Si le rétablissement des sciences et des arts a contribué à pururer les mœurs." This would lay the foundations of his famous and polemical discourse on sciences and arts. This was the form in which open challenges took place. Some of them date back to 1714 when the government of England offered £20,000 to anyone who could accurately calculate the longitudinal position of a ship.

If the mastery of writing or calculation acts as a natural, census-based filter, then the idea of opening up participation in a competition to any candidate regardless of any institutional affiliation is the thread that open science is reviving today. Global connection to the internet, the availability of general knowledge (particularly, through Wikipedia[4]), free access to hard science articles via Arxiv,[5] the democratization of access to advanced technological resources (notably, via open-source tools) all nowadays provide the means of building a more open, inclusive science able to complement academic expertise with the contributions of collective intelligence and to increase the creative production of the former by a certain spirit of disruption whose likelihood we postulate here is freely distributed among the population.

## From Microtasking to Challenges

Open science distinguishes two sources of benefits derived from reasonable mobilization of collective intelligence. On the one hand, the mass effect ensures the execution of simple but massive tasks by distributing them in a so-called microtasking network. An example is the Stardust@home[6] project initiated by NASA, which asks volunteer to detect traces of dust impacting on the Stardust space probe using a virtual microscope. The idea was to parallelize an elementary task that would leave a handful of individuals demoralized by the scale of it. Stardust@home will in turn inspire one of the most famous collaborative projects called Zooniverse,[7] which consists in bringing together hundreds of thousands of people to classify the shape of galaxies on the basis of telescopic images.

Another way of involving everyone in science is through challenges that are sometimes more complex.

Using resources that collective intelligence offers in the field of health is no longer an advocacy issue having now become the reality of new approaches. Analysis of the medical scientific literature shows that since the beginning of this decade public health research or cancer research has intensified the use of such approaches. For the most part, these are the implications of performing data analysis from its solicitation through questionnaires to mobilization around complex problems taking on the form

---

[4]https://www.wikipedia.org/.

[5]https://arxiv.org/.

[6]http://stardustathome.ssl.berkeley.edu/.

[7]https://www.zooniverse.org/.

of challenges. We will give various examples illustrating different facets of scientific knowledge found in the interactions between academic and informal environments:

- *Cooperation*—In 2013 the Sage Bionetworks[8] team and its partners mobilized hundreds of citizens and researchers for a period of six months. The subject matter was the predictability of breast cancer and the project was called the Digital Mammography DREAM Challenge.[9] The aim was to evaluate through this community challenge the practice of open, citizen-based science to improve prognostic reference models. Moreover, this turned out to be the case so much so that today Sage Bionetworks operates many seminal challenges (particularly, in the field of cancer) and in so doing ensures the development of open science while consolidating its approaches.
- *Heterodoxy*—In attempts to understand protein plicature (i.e., folding), which gives it its functional properties, researchers at the University of Washington have invited internet users to play at bending proteins through a playful interface. The Foldit[10] project in a unique way will have rewarded researchers as a result of unaware people making use of knowledge in molecular biology and even helped researchers understand the role of certain proteins involved in HIV.
- *Open source*—Competitions such as IGEM[11] or Epidemium[12] enable many competitors to come up with original solutions in the fields of synthetic biology or cancer research based on open data. These are communities of diverse origins and heterogeneous profiles that get to know each other, share their knowledge, and form multidisciplinary teams to develop technological tools for research and other solutions for health professionals and patients. This production of content, whether originating from algorithms or cleansed databases, published under open licenses makes it possible for anyone to distribute, audit, use, and improve them thus fostering interplay of a broad, potentially global collaboration.

Thus, a large number of projects documenting what could be called "gray literature" are led by open communities primarily developing generic instruments that can be reused in many fields such as biology, physics, and informatics.

# Epidemium

Born out of a meeting between the community laboratory La Paillasse and the pharmaceutical company Roche France in 2015, the Epidemium program is defined as a newly distributed research framework. Dedicated to understanding cancer through

---

[8]http://sagebionetworks.org/.

[9]https://www.synapse.org/#!Synapse:syn4224222/wiki/401743.

[10]https://fold.it/portal/.

[11]http://igem.org/Main_Page.

[12]http://epidemium.cc/.

open data and Big Data technologies it is based on openness, collaboration, and knowledge sharing.

## Definition of the Program

Epidemium is positioned as a neutral third space (both virtual and physical) and as a catalyst promoting synergies capable of welcoming not just traditional research actors, but also more broadly all those interested in the problem of cancer epidemiology whatever their nature, their field, and level of expertise to enable them to advance research together. From patients, to doctors, and to all data specialists—any individual can come to this shared environment to discuss, develop a common culture and language, and exchange and understand different points of view.

More concretely, by the end of 2017 Epidemium had brought together a transdisciplinary community (data scientists, doctors, patients, researchers, sociologists, graphic designers, etc.) exceeding 1200 people, building an ecosystem of several hundred experts, and a network of involved partners who provide participants with technical, material, and human resources. It also has an independent ethics committee and a scientific committee composed of recognized personalities from the world of medical research and data science who support the program in its design and implementation and guide participants in their work.

All these actors are united by the desire to address the major challenges facing research on this pathology and to prototype solutions to:

- share resources, expertise, and achievements to code to develop scientific knowledge;
- explore new avenues of cancer research within a methodological and ethical framework;
- accelerate research by taking advantage of collective intelligence and rapid prototyping; and
- improve existing assumptions and solutions using the potential of open source and Big Data technologies.

## A Framework for Scientific Cooperation

From an organizational point of view Epidemium operates its research program in the form of six-month challenges that are open to all. The program's themes are based on cancer epidemiology. This has made it possible to develop a logic of collaboration and competition to stimulate all stakeholders and to enable the transdisciplinary community to work together to propose innovative and complementary approaches to traditional research.

All individuals regardless of their skills and areas of expertise are invited to come and discover the program and possibly contribute according to their availability and will. Epidemium community productions are developed under open licenses so that they are freely accessible and can be circulated, taken up by all, and improved for the ultimate benefit of all.

Although the ultimate objective is to demonstrate that a collaborative and open program is capable of producing scientific knowledge and getting published, there are other aims:

- aggregating, cleansing, and matching public data from a set of open data platforms made available to participants and associated with analysis environments;
- providing platforms bringing together all program participants and projects, and integrating various tools to support teamwork (Wiki, GitLab, RocketChat, OwnCloud);
- sharing resources, expertise, and achievements to code and develop scientific knowledge;
- providing events in several formats (meetups, training, acceleration day, etc.) to meet different objectives such as acculturation, training, support, and acceleration of projects; and
- Giving honorary mentions (by the committees constituted as a jury at the end of the challenges) to distinguish the projects according to several criteria such as patient health, ethics, data visualization, Wiki, originality, collaboration, and proposals for a scientific article.

In this way projects of world renown and global scope have been codeveloped by communities and published in open source such as the Raspberry Py[13] computer or the Arduino[14] microcontroller (hardware) and R or latex (software). Such projects are providing science with powerful statistical analysis tools and other scientific editing tools and are serving in turn as a starting point for new projects thus strengthening the conduct of open, inclusive, and collaborative science.

Although many projects are born thanks to the spontaneous organization of communities of individuals, it should be noted that the scaling up of these dynamics and the production of truly usable "scalable" solutions presupposes the potentialization of cocreative dynamics by sustainable and supported organizations. In the projects mentioned subsequently it should be noted that projects such as Linux or R are structured by foundations receiving sustainable funding.

## Central Resource: Open Data

The primary raw material related to these new approaches is open data. Open data, the resource made available by the promoters of this collaborative science, make it

---

[13]https://www.raspberrypi.org/.

[14]https://www.arduino.cc/.

possible for a larger number of interested parties to invite themselves into research fields that are sometimes compartmentalized in narrowly institutional circuits. After having fallen behind the Anglo-Saxon countries in implementing an open-data strategy, France has become one of the leading and most advanced productive countries on the subject. This dynamic began at the start of the 2010s with the establishment of EtaLab, France's dedicated political innovation laboratory, and the website data. gouv.fr[15] that collects and publicly displays open-data games produced by the central administration and local authorities. Thus, in just a few years France has become a model nation in the field of open data, as shown by its ranking in the Open Data Index produced annually by the Open Knowledge Foundation[16] that ranks France in fourth place among nations promoting open data. The political climate of appropriating open-data challenges is therefore entirely conducive to the emergence of such a strong dynamic in the field of open science in France.

## Open Science, Open Data, and Reproducibility in Life Sciences

At another level the use of open data in science that is more inclusive can enhance traditional science as a result of new better quality contributions (especially, in the field of life sciences). Indeed, in addition to the greater inclusiveness promoted by an open-data culture a crucial issue enters the debate on the release of open data: that of the quality of research and its reproducibility in which the notion of data sharing and transparency plays a decisive role. Indeed, life sciences place reproducibility at the heart of their epistemology. The results of an experiment are only claimed if they can be reproduced. This is the benefit of open data since they allow any third party to verify the results claimed by authors. Moreover, open data are not in themselves new but represent the emergence of a practice that is common in many other scientific fields.

This is dogged by a problem that dominates the production of knowledge in the life sciences as a whole even beyond the perspectives that new technologies offer: the remarkably low reproducibility of results in biomedical research. This field of investigation, sometimes referred to as research on research, estimates that the rate of irreproducibility of biomedical research is around 70% according to recent publications. The reasons for these poor results are wide-ranging and difficulties in accessing data partly reflect this. Indeed, even today authors are not required to share their data so that their analysis can be checked and reproduced.

Of course, the first obstacle is the sensitive nature of personal data prohibiting their publication. Then there is the major interest in developing techniques to prevent data deanonymization to improve transparency and the quality of results, a research area involving many teams in computer science and mathematics. The notion of

---

[15]https://www.data.gouv.fr/.
[16]https://okfn.org/.

differential privacy has thus recently been conceptualized providing a mathematical formulation for the "privacy" of data and a means of attaching a metric to it. It is therefore reasonable to think that in the coming years anonymization techniques will appear that will allow the release of non-reidentifying open data datasets for the greater benefit of the auditability of research results and, ultimately, the quality of production conditions. A singular example is the use of artificial intelligence techniques for data simulation purposes and real-data datasets allowing algorithms to learn to locate patterns, then be returned in a simulated dataset that is by definition anonymized, and finally presented in the form of open data.

## Open Source: The Cornerstone of an Open Model

Open source, whether in the development of software or hardware, is taking on ever more importance as a coconstruction approach to solutions thus allowing the interests of players to converge and resources to pool. Today the National Institute of Health (NIH) increasingly requires code to be open-sourced when funding projects. The Bill and Melinda Gates Foundation does the same by requesting that all the work it takes on be published in open access and the results given open licenses.

This approach allows for more inclusive development, on the one hand, and a real pooling of development capacities, funds, resources, and assets that everyone can reuse, on the other hand.

New economic models are gradually emerging from this dynamic in terms of putting a value on cocreated assets using licenses allowing free use of solutions when it comes to community or academic practices and paid use when it comes to commercial reuse. Basically, the open-source business model is "spending time to save money versus spending money to save time."

All in all, we are on the verge of developing new and pioneering ways of doing science. Conservatism is all that stands in the way of scientific revocation. This is not the result of the discovery of new planets, new drugs, or new theorems, but the discovery by the scientific community of new actors recognized as legitimate and just as powerful as any of us. By conservatism we mean those who would deny access to science from a public well versed and authorized on titles and works, as well as those who are prisoners of an ideology closed to openness and who would see in the academy a dusty old-fashioned, state-subsidized phenomenon. The important thing is to articulate these two worlds. We can rejoice that the meeting places are multiple, which bodes well for a paradigmatic break in the ways knowledge is produced.

It is therefore necessary to maintain public efforts to open up public data because, let's face it, it would be counterintuitive if public data were not available to the public.

# Data

# Data: Protection and Legal Conditions of Access and Processing

**Jeanne Bossi-Malafosse**

Personal data are the raw material of media research and the basis of Big Data. The capabilities offered by artificial intelligence techniques make the conditions for data collection and processing even more essential.

The French Data Protection Act has so far provided the essential legal framework for the processing of personal data. Today it must comply with the new European Data Protection Regulation of April 27, 2016 and adapt to allow Big Data to develop for the benefit of public health.

The legal conditions for the processing of health data at the time of entry into force of the European Regulation will be presented in this chapter together with the view of the Commission Nationale de l'Informatique et des Libertés (CNIL).

The chapter will also illustrate what can be achieved today by a health data analysis company and why Big Data and data protection are not incompatible.

Since May 25, 2018 the collection and processing of personal health data has been subject to conditions laid down in the European Data Protection Regulation of April 27, 2016. They have to be deployed in a complex and changing national legal context that is supposed to be able to meet the challenges of Big Data.

General Data Protection Regulations (GDPRs)[1] have therefore been applicable since May 25, 2018. They introduce new concepts and modify the obligations of actors involved in the processing of personal data. Their objectives are multiple such as replacing the 1995 Directive, strengthening the rights of individuals, and ensuring homogeneous and consistent application of rules on the protection of personal data.

---

[1] See in this respect Recital 53 of the EU General Data Protection Regulation (RGPD).

---

J. Bossi-Malafosse (✉)
Personal Data and Health Information Systems, DELSOL Avocats, Paris, France
e-mail: jbossimalafosse@delsolavocats.com

© Springer Nature Switzerland AG 2020
B. Nordlinger et al. (eds.), *Healthcare and Artificial Intelligence*,
https://doi.org/10.1007/978-3-030-32161-1_28

The Regulations establish the principle of accountability under which each actor must be able to prove at all times that processing operations carried out comply with the principles of personal data protection. Combined with the obligation to integrate upstream of all projects the principles of data protection (i.e., privacy by design) the Regulations introduce a new approach to the protection of personal data.

While this new European text has an impact on all activities, it recognizes that some data "deserve higher protection" such as health and genetic data. Their processing is subject to the provisions of the Regulations, but Member States have room to maneuver to maintain or introduce "additional conditions including limitations as regards the processing of genetic data, biometric data or health data"[2] thus reflecting various health organizations.

Integrating the new principles laid down by the Regulations and exercising this room for maneuver have required adapting the previous French Data Protection Act.[3] A new law on data protection was adopted in June 2018 and rewritten in December 2018 to adapt national law to the European text and came into force in June 2019 (hereinafter the new law).

The processing of health data must therefore incorporate today the provisions of the GDPR, those of Law No. 78–17 of January 6, 1978 on data processing, files, and freedoms (hereinafter the Data Protection Act), and its amendment with the adoption of the new law. It must also take into account all the provisions of the Public Health Code and the Social Security Code that may impact their collection and processing.

At a time when Big Data, understood here as the ability to process ever-increasing quantities of data from a wide variety of sources, is being developed it is essential to adapt the legal framework.

# Impact of EU General Data Protection Regulations on the Processing of Health Data

## Definition of Health Data and Appropriate Safeguards

The EU GDPRs provide a new definition of health data. They define health data as all information relating to the identification of the patient in the healthcare system or device used to collect and process health data, all information obtained during a medical examination or control including biological samples, genomic data, and all medical information. For example, diseases; handicaps; risks for disease; clinical, therapeutic, physiological, or biological data regardless of their source whether coming from doctors, other health professionals, medical devices, or in vivo or in vitro explorations.[4]

---

[2]Ibid.

[3]Law No. 78–17 of January 6, 1978 amended on information technology, files, and freedoms.

[4]See EP and Cons. EU, Reg. (EU) No. 2016/679, April 27, 2016, Recital 35.

This new definition reflects a broader concept of health data taking into account that patients' healthcare also requires knowledge of their family or social situation and involves multiple actors, health professionals, and social personnel.

This broadened concept of health data is in line with the redefined notion of the healthcare team in France by Act No. 2016-41 of January 26, 2016, which brings together "a group of professionals who participate directly for the benefit of the same patient in the performance of a diagnostic, therapeutic, disability compensation, pain managment or prevention of loss of independance, or in the actions necessary for [their] coordination."[5]

Health data are therefore considered by the GDPRs[6] and the Data Protection Act[7] as sensitive data whose processing should be subject to special protection.

## Principle of Prohibition with Derogations

Like Articles 6 and 44 of the Data Protection Act, the GDPRs lay down the principle of prohibiting the processing of sensitive data.[8]

This principle is accompanied by a series of exceptions (derogations) allowing them to be processed. This Regulation is subject to the following exceptions: the explicit consent of the person (unless the law of a Member State or the Union provides that the prohibition cannot be lifted by such consent alone); the enforcement of obligations or rights in the field of social protection; protection of the vital interests of the person; the legitimate interest of the data controller who determine the purpose and the means of the collection of data with appropriate safeguards; on the grounds of public interest and all necessary processing operations for the purposes of preventive or occupational medicine, medical diagnosis, health or social care, or the management of health or social protection systems and services.[9]

This Regulation also allows the processing of sensitive data for reasons of public interest in the field of public health or for the purpose of ensuring high standards of quality and safety of healthcare, medicinal products, and medical devices, as well as for scientific research.

---

[5] Article L.1110-12 of the Public Health Code. This broad understanding of the health sector integrating the health, medicosocial, or social sector is also reflected in the Council of Europe's draft recommendation on health data published in 2018.

[6] Article 9 of the GDPRs.

[7] Article 6 and 44 of the French Data Protection Act.

[8] Reg. (EU) No. 2016/679, April 27, 2016, Recital 10.

[9] For an exhaustive list see Article 9§2, EP and Cons. EU, Reg. (EU) No. 2016/679, April 27, 2016.

> ## Chapter IX of the French Data Protection Act, tomorrow
>
> The new law on data protection aimed at adapting the Data Protection Act to the GDPRs chooses to bring together in the same Chapter IX all processing of personal health data for whatever purpose.
>
> It introduces as a single and common criterion for all processing of health data the notion of public interest except in the cases referred to in 10 to 60 of draft Article 8-II and processing operations enabling studies to be carried out on the basis of data collected in the context of the administration of care pursuant to 60 of II of Article 8 when such studies are carried out by monitoring staff and intended for their exclusive use; processing carried out for the purpose of ensuring the provision of benefits or supervision by compulsory and supplementary health insurance bodies; processing carried out within health establishments by doctors responsible for medical information; processing carried out by regional health agencies, by the State, and by the public person designated by it pursuant to the first paragraph of Article L.6113-8 of the Public Health Code.

While this orientation is understandable and may serve the purpose of clarification, the choice to treat all processing operations under the same single section entitled "General Provisions," whether it is a matter of providing care or conducting research, is likely to introduce confusion and lead to governments imposing obligations on the former that are characteristic of the latter.

Draft Article 54 maintains a cumbersome system of prior formalities (authorization) since its processing cannot be certified as being in conformity with standard reference systems and regulations established by the CNIL in consultation with the Institut national des données de santé, which contradicts the spirit of relief provided by the Regulation.

As is the case of personal data of any kind, the processing of health data must comply with lawfulness conditions laid down by the GDPRs and the controller must implement technical and organizational measures to ensure compliance with the principles of personal data protection.

## Compatibility of Personal Data Protection Principles with the Development of Big Data

Any use of health data must comply with the five main principles of personal data protection as put forward by the GDPRs.

> **The five principles of personal data protection**
>
> – Determined, explicit, and legitimate processing purpose
> – Adequate and relevant data (minimization principle)
> – Fixed storage period
> – Respect for the rights of individuals regarding information and, where applicable, consent
> – Security measures to ensure data confidentiality.

All actors using health data must be able to prove at all times that the processing operations they are implementing comply with these principles (accountability). Associated with the obligation to integrate data protection principles (privacy by design), accountability introduces a new approach to the protection of personal data.

The processing of health data is not excluded from this new way of managing data protection as shown by the fact that impact studies to analyze risks to fundamental rights and freedoms are required for large-scale processing of health data.[10]

In addition to elements such as these that are common to personal data processing of all kinds, it is interesting to note that the Regulations contain certain provisions that appear new and may be useful in the age of new data-mining techniques (particularly, those used in the context of Big Data and artificial intelligence). For example, the GDPRs introduce the notion of purpose compatible with the purpose for which the data were collected, which is likely to facilitate the reuse of data when they have been collected in a lawful manner without weakening the rights of individuals.

When it comes to the nature of the data collected the GDPRs enshrine the concept of pseudonymization.[11] Even if pseudonymized data remain personal data, they can still facilitate data collection in cases where the collection of directly named data would have been more complicated.

When it comes to the rights of individuals the GDPRs make it possible to relax the obligation to inform the data subject in certain specific cases. This is particularly the case when "the provision of such information proves impossible or would require disproportionate efforts" subject to the adoption of appropriate measures to protect the rights, freedoms, and legitimate interests of the person concerned. This provision is particularly useful in research investigating the possibility of secondary use of data and in cases where it would be too constraining to find the person to inform him or her.[12]

---

[10]Section 35 of the RGPD.

[11]Article 4 of the RGPD defines pseudonymization as "the processing of personal data in such a way that they can no longer be attributed to a specific data subject without recourse to additional information, provided that this additional information is kept separately and subject to technical and organisational measures to ensure that personal data are not attributed to an identified or identifiable natural person.".

[12]Automated decision-making is then only possible with the consent of the person concerned, on the grounds of public interest, or provided that appropriate measures to safeguard the rights and freedoms and legitimate interests of the person concerned are not in place.

Concerned with achieving a characteristic balance in the text the GDPRs strengthen the rights of data subjects in the face of the use of new data analysis techniques. The data subject shall have the right not to be subject to a decision based solely on automated processing, including profiling, which produces legal effects concerning him or her or similarly significantly affects him or her. This right is more strictly applied when it concerns sensitive data including health data. The notion of clearly identified profiling will therefore need to be assessed at the time of algorithm development.

When it comes to data security, a major aspect of the text, the GDPRs state that it should be adapted to the sensitive nature of the data (risk analysis) and that the application of soft law tools (code of conduct, certification) may be used to demonstrate compliance with security requirements.

It should be noted that the new French law gives the CNIL the possibility to establish and publish model regulations to ensure the security of personal data–processing systems and to regulate the processing of health data covered by Chapter IX.[13]

The new obligation to notify a data breach where it is likely to create a risk to the rights and freedoms of individuals is in line with the obligation provided for[14] by the Public Health Code that requires healthcare institutions, organizations, and services engaged in prevention, diagnosis, or care activities to report health information system security incidents to ASIP Santé (French Agency of Numerical Health).[15]

To ensure the implementation of these principles and compliance with them the appointment of a data protection officer (DPO) is mandatory for controllers and processors carrying out large-scale processing of sensitive data (in particular, health data).[16]

In addition to all these requirements there are Regulations that are not just specific to health data in France, they also illustrate the room for maneuver of Member States.

---

[13] The CNIL had already anticipated these principles by drafting reference methods that put in place minimum safety measures and involve carrying out risk analysis that prefigures conduct of the impact study required by the Regulations.

[14] Article 33 of the GDPRs.

[15] Article L.1111-8-2 of the Public Health Code stipulates that "Health establishments and bodies and services carrying out prevention, diagnosis or care activities shall report serious incidents of information system security to the regional health agency without delay. Safety incidents deemed significant are also transmitted without delay by the regional health agency to the competent State authorities.".

[16] Reg. (EU) No. 2016/679, April 27, 2016, Article 39(2).

# Room for Maneuver Left to National Law: High Level of Security in a Complex Legal Environment

## *Exchange and Sharing of Health Data*

The processing of personal health data as defined in the GDPRs is part of a legal framework in France provided for by the Public Health Code. These provisions were recently renewed by the adoption of Act No. 2016-41 of January 26, 2016 on modernization of the French health system.

The new definition of health data proposed by the Regulations should be read by taking into consideration the notion of a care team now redefined and adapted to the reality of sharing personal data. To this end the new Article L.1110-4 of the Public Health Code, while reaffirming secrecy, redefines the regime for the exchange and sharing of personal health data by articulating it with a broader notion of the healthcare team.

This new definition of the care team is associated with an harmonization of information and consent of patients concerned. Among the care team, the patient must received a prior information about their right but do not have to consent to share their data, the consent of the person being reserved for the sharing of information outside the care team.

These provisions are important because they facilitate the collection of data that can be used for research purposes. Article L.1110-4-1 of the Public Health Code[17] refers to the obligation of information system managers to comply with safety and interoperability guidelines defined by ASIP Santé and approved by an order issued by the Minister of Health (after consulting the CNIL) and published in the *Official Journal*.

---

### Security and interoperability standards

- *Certification of the identity of health professionals involved in information systems—Shared Directory of Health Professionals (RPPS)—and the assignment of appropriate means of authentication.*
- *Patient identity certification to ensure identity vigilance within information systems: the social security number is the national health identifier (NHI).*
- *The certification of providers of personal health data.*
- *The national framework for the interoperability of information systems (technical and semantic interoperability).*

---

[17] Article L.1110-12 of the Public Health Code.

## *Reuse of Health Data*

A complex and currently evolving legal framework governs the conditions of access to health data for research. It involves implementing the principles of the GDPRs, the Data Protection Act, and the new law on data protection (the new law) amending the previous Data Protection Act.

The conditions that need to be met to process data for research purposes are currently referred to in Chapter IX of the Data Protection Act (Articles 53 et seq.) and define a self-regulation regime for all processing of personal data for the purposes of research, study, or evaluation in the health sector. This procedure must be read in conjunction with the provisions of Article 193 of the law of January 26, 2016 on modernization of the French health system, which also creates a new legal regime for access to medical and administrative databases with the creation of the National System of Health Data (NSHD), composed of the major medical and administrative databases.[18]

The conditions that need to be met to gain access to the NSHD NSHDS[19] are limited to:

- study, or evaluation purposes contributing to a purpose mentioned in III of Article L.1461-1 of the Public Health Code[20] and responding to a reason in the public interest;
- performance of tasks laid down by government departments, public institutions, or bodies responsible for a public service mission (i.e., a specific access procedure for organizations with a public service mission).

The procedure referred to in the last bullet involves the new National Institute for Health Data (INDS)[21] and the Committee of Expertise for Research, Studies and Evaluation in the Field of Health (CEREES). The latter decides which methodology

---

[18]SNIIRAM (data from the social security sytem), PMSI (data from hospitals), medical causes of death, CNSA (data from the social system).

[19]Decree No. 2016-1871 of December 26, 2016 on the processing of personal data referred to as NHDS SDS.

[20]According to II the purpose of the national health data system is to make the data under conditions defined in Articles L.1461-2 and L.1461-3 available and to contribute to information on health and on the provision of care, medicosocial care, and its quality; the definition, implementation, and evaluation of health and social protection policies; to knowledge about health expenses, health insurance expenses, and medicosocial expenses; informing health or medicosocial professionals, structures, and institutions about their activity; health monitoring, surveillance, and safety; research, studies, evaluation, and innovation in the fields of health and medicosocial care.

[21]The public interest group INDS was created by decree on April 20, 2017 and has the following missions: ensuring the quality of health data and the general conditions under which they are made available, guaranteeing their security, and facilitating their use; providing a single window for requests for access to data for research purposes; issuing opinions on the public interest nature of research, studies, or evaluations; facilitating the availability of samples or approved datasets mentioned in conditions previously approved by the CNIL; and contributing to dialogue on the need for anonymous data and statistical results with a view to making them available to the public.

is adopted, the need for personal data to be used, their relevance to the purpose pursued, and where appropriate the scientific status of the project.[22]

This recently introduced procedure raises questions of a different nature relating to the complexity, the more restrictive regime imposed on private actors, and the offbeat approach to stakeholder accountability put forward by the GDPRs.

In addition to this there is the regulatory framework for research involving human beings, recently reviewed by the Jardé Act, which must also be integrated into the authorization system of Articles 65 et seq. of the Data Protection Act.[23]

The notion of public interest, which does not have any precise legal definition, introduces subjectivity into assessing such interest and legitimate concern on the part of stakeholders who are concerned about the importance now given it. Such concern was not previously there when assessing how a research project complies with rules on the protection of personal data.

The flexible way this concept, recently introduced by the CNIL, can be interpreted when it comes to health data warehouses, whether conducted by public or private organizations, must be maintained to allow the development of Big Data[24] tools.

However, it seems that these fears were heard by Parliament in the context of discussions on the bill to adapt to the GDPRs, which now take into account alongside the public interest purpose the other purpose provided for in the Regulations such as protecting against serious cross-border threats to health or ensuring high standards of quality and safety of health care and of medicinal products or medical devices.

All these developments should facilitate access to health data while respecting human rights. However, such developments must also be accompanied by policies aimed at organizing the IT systems in such a way that in addition to the production function of care a knowledge production function contributes to raising the standards of public health.

---

[22]This committee is an offshoot of the Advisory Committee on the Processing of Health Research Information and has similar missions.

[23]Fortunately, the CNIL can simplify reference methodologies and single authorizations as long as it has already made use of them.

[24]Deliberations Nos. 2017-013 and 2017–285.

The principles underlying personal data protection remain essential legal and ethical references in a State governed by the rule of law. EU Regulation through its territorial application criteria now creates Europe-wide protection that is binding even on entities outside its territory where persons living on the territory of the Union are concerned.

However, at a time when our societies are being "datafied" (particularly, in the health sector) with the new analytical capabilities that characterize Big Data, it is imperative that data protection principles be interpreted with pragmatism and flexibility. We know that the new European text gives us the opportunity to do so by, for example, outlining purposes that are compatible and conditions that are necessary for reidentification. However, it will be the decision of politicians voting on the texts and how they should be interpreted by authorities tasked with protecting personal data and organizations that intervene in the procedures provided for by the Data Protection Act that will enable both to use the data available and to respect personal rights.

There must be no conflict between the protection of rights and public health objectives that today require the massive collection and use of personal data. The protection of rights must not be used by some to reflect reluctance or even in some cases a lost attempt to maintain power in advance over data that are not subject to ownership because they are considered human attributes.

# CNIL (Commission Nationale de l'Informatique et des Libertés) and Analysis of Big Data Projects in the Health Sector

Matthieu Grall

## Context and Issues

We hear a lot about Big Data. Everyone talks about Big Data and everyone has an opinion on the issue—such opinions as "Big Data is the engine that consumes the oil of personal data," "Too many Big Data algorithms provide answers very precisely to the wrong questions or to unauthorized data," "GAFAs know more about us than insurers," "Big Data can quickly impact ethics," and "Personal data protection is the ethical safeguard of Big Data."

Generally speaking, when it comes to processing personal data based on Big Data the main risks are the misuse of data (especially, concerning privacy), processing (automated decisions and difficulty or even impossibility to exercise rights of access, rights to rectification, and rights to object), and finally the data themselves (secret collection, lack of information or consent about how collected, unreliability of the data, confusion between the public and private spheres, difficulty or even impossibility to set retention periods or to delete data at the end of their retention period).

But are we always talking about the same thing? Uses differ when it comes to rapid analysis of massive and heterogeneous data made possible by new storage and processing technologies.

## Toward a Finer Typology of Adapted Solutions

Distinctions should be made between the types of processing based on Big Data so that possibilities for their use can be identified and managed appropriately.

M. Grall (✉)

Department of the Commission Nationale de l'Informatique et des Libertés, Paris, France

e-mail: mgrall@cnil.fr

A first criterion for making distinctions could be the origin of data. Five cases can be identified: clinical or experimental data, pharmaceutical databases, open data, data from connected objects, and patient data. Data are normally collected by organizations (direct collection or reuse of data for other purposes) but there are exceptions (public external data or pooling of several sources).

A second criterion for making distinctions could be the general objective of processing that can be broken down into two main categories: the detection of trends (e.g., to identify a phenomenon or to produce statistics) and predictive targeting of a person (e.g., to find information on someone identified or to identify someone on the basis of information).

By combining these two sets of criteria eight cases can be distinguished as illustrated by some examples of health data processing in Table 1.

**Table 1** Typology and examples in the health field

| | Object | |
|---|---|---|
| Source | Detection of trends | Targeting of a person/survey on a person/prediction with identification |
| Direct collection | Contribute to a specific research project | Diagnose a pathology or adapt an individual therapeutic strategy (decision support) |
| | | Perform self-measurements and restore them |
| Reuse of data for other purposes | Contribute to other research projects | Obtain an overview by correlating data to improve practices |
| | Effectiveness of the health system, health monitoring | Perform simulations on the basis of real cases (pedagogy) |
| External Public Data | Carry out vigilance studies (pharmacology, materials, infections vigilance) | Carry out targeted vigilance studies (pharmacology, materials, infection vigilance) |
| | Contribute to research | Diagnose a pathology or adapt a therapeutic strategy (decision support) |
| | | Detect risky behaviors (social networks) |
| Pooling of several sources | Obtain an overview by correlating data to improve practices | Obtain an overview of an individual case by correlating data to assist in the decision |
| | Perform simulations on the basis of real cases (pedagogy) | |

Such cases facilitate understanding contexts and in so doing anticipate and deal more precisely with the risks that each of the cases entails for the rights and freedoms of the persons concerned.

For example, the processing of public external data to detect trends could be based on legitimate interests in which there is no decision-making or individualized feedback. Alternately, just open data could be processed. Another example would be the processing of data compiled for a targeted purpose, which could be based on consent or a legal basis or be subject to authorization or advice by authorities, and which would implement such mechanisms as transparency and portability.

Finally, anonymization could also be considered in some cases. If datasets are genuinely anonymized the General Data Protection Regulations (GDPRs) no longer apply. However, anonymization is very difficult to set up.

## *Big Data* and Anonymization of Data, How to Reconcile Them?

The GDPR[1] links the notion of anonymous data to "means reasonably likely to be used" to re-identify the persons concerned.

This is therefore based on a logic of re-identification risks. And it quickly becomes apparent that the tools used to materialize these risks are quite similar to those of Big Data. Indeed, researchers who have studied these risks on *open-data* sets have used the following techniques

- cross-referencing with more identifying data sources;
- internal correlation of the data, enabling to find the various records related to the same person;
- inferences that make it possible for additional characteristics to be deduced about a given person.

From a different angle, it appears that these techniques, which carry the expected results of a Big Data approach, are exactly orthogonal to the data anonymization criteria defined by the WP29[2]! It could almost be said that Big Data, by its mode of operation, interferes with the anonymization of the data.

So, is it possible to do Big Data on anonymous data? Yes, provided that data impoverishment (inherent in meeting the WP29 criteria) is properly targeted to retain only the data elements that are to be used. This requires a preliminary study and implementation for a specific purpose.[3]

Finally, there is the case of "data *mining*" (*data mining, deep learning, etc.*), which requires both a large amount of information and very precise elements, without having a prior definition of what is precisely being sought. In fact, the data used will then be difficult to "anonymize according to the WP29 criteria" and will at most be "pseudonymized" or "de-identified" in order not to keep direct identifiers of persons (surname, date and place of birth, etc.).

This case is also the most risky in terms of the results of algebraic algorithms, which may have categorized people and made inferences about sensitive characteristics (health status, sexual orientation, religion, etc.). It will then be necessary to protect access to the raw results and to work on making them anonymous in order to make them publishable.

In summary and in practice, unless prior and active work is carried out to preserve the anonymization of the data throughout its processing, Big Data will be considered as processing personal data and will therefore have to comply with their protection by the GDPR.

---

1. GDPR, recital 26.
2. Opinion 05/2014 on Anonymisation Techniques, 0829/14/FR WP216, Article 29 Working Party.
3. Cabanon, Orange.

## Objective: To Develop Understanding and Trust

If Big Data are really going to deliver the enormous potential they have for new services in the health sector, taking privacy into account now appears to be the sine qua non solution to bring about trust when it comes to users and patients. In a context where everything is revealed, threats are real, and technology sometimes passes us by this need for trust becomes an essential issue. Using the GDPRs the CNIL wishes to move forward with actors in the health sector to develop a pragmatic doctrine.

The objective now is to refine typologies (in particular, the types of purposes) and the way each case is treated. Typologies should also be refined to treat specific contexts such as non-perennial experiments, pseudonymized data, connected objects, and artificial intelligence. This can be done by testing typologies and studying more and more real cases, say, in the form of data protection impact assessments more commonly known as privacy impact assessments (PIAs) that take into account the whole of the data life cycle, from collection to storage, modeling, analysis, use, and eventual destruction.

Therefore, there is a need to identify and study specific projects of all kinds to generalize the various problems encountered and adapt solutions to them. In this way requests for advice may enable those wishing to implement projects based on Big Data to work with the CNIL.

# International Vision of Big Data

**Laurent Degos**

All countries, even the poorest, are moving toward digital technology. The digital revolution in health is taking place more or less rapidly depending on the nation. It disrupts the practice and organization of care in advanced countries or facilitates it in emerging countries. Digital technology is being introduced at the same pace as it is being accepted by the population. Between reluctance to change and the attraction of innovation for faster access to care the radical digital divide is not without its challenges.[1]

Two main areas of digital technology are transforming the health system: (1) technological tools to assist care (telemedicine, medical applications on smartphones, connected objects, sensors, robots, etc.) that pose problems when it comes to evaluating their benefits and potential reimbursement for their use and (2) mass data opening the way to artificial intelligence through deep learning.

Although the former can be included in known schemes to evaluate medical technologies and compare values (benefit/risk, utility, etc.) for individual use, the latter require other financing, other values, and other levers for collective benefit that is still unclear and poorly defined.

This second aspect (i.e., the collection of mass data, their analysis, and the applications they enable) is the subject of this review of progress in various countries. We will use major themes to make comparisons and describe examples of advanced countries in terms of the mass data digitized in this chapter and not through a country-by-country review.

---

[1]International reflection on Big Data was recently conducted by the Commonwealth Fund in April 2016 (Washington), by the Scientific Panel for Health (SPH of the European Commission's DG RTD (Directotate General for reseach and innovation, European commission)) in June 2017 (Brussels), and … by the Care Insight symposium "Health and Tech for People" in December 2017 (Paris). This chapter was inspired by these reflections.

---

L. Degos (✉)
Academy of Medicine, Academy of Sciences, University of Paris, Paris, France
e-mail: laurentdegos@gmail.com

© Springer Nature Switzerland AG 2020
B. Nordlinger et al. (eds.), *Healthcare and Artificial Intelligence*,
https://doi.org/10.1007/978-3-030-32161-1_30

The WHO through its e-Health Observatory has calculated that 17% of countries have a policy on Big Data in the health sector. The World Bank finds a similar percentage that is practically identical in poor countries (16%), developing countries (14%), and rich countries (23%).

Several types of health databases have been established since the onset of the digital revolution including medical records; administrative data; insurance data; and data collected from connected objects, cohorts, registers, death certificates, surveys, social networks, genomic data, etc. In fact, medical records represent the most exploited source and the greatest difficulty is making links between multiple databases.

The thinking in each country is based on the assumption that the amount of data collected makes it possible to detect weak signals that are invisible in therapeutic trials, to evaluate a practice or product in real life, to prospectively monitor the spread of a phenomenon such as an epidemic, and to reveal unknown correlations (data mining). However, correlation does not mean a cause-and-effect relationship.

Big Data also open the way for machine learning to clarify diagnosis and decision-making as experience increases. Currently, this field of exploration (i.e., artificial intelligence in health) is mainly applied to imaging and epidemiology.

Some countries such as Estonia are strongly committed to digital technology; others are making digital means of collecting data from media files obligatory as stipulated in the US Health Information Technology for Economic and Clinical Health (HITECH) Act; yet others such as France insist on privacy because the analysis of personal data requires abandoning a certain amount of confidentiality.

There is also the question of the role played by public authorities (NHS in England) or the private sector (Kaiser Permanente in the United States) in the collection, analysis, and application of large health databases.

All countries today recognize the value of digital technology and realize that value is not so much financial as societal modifying the paradigm of health value (price and reimbursement). New values are considered such as equality, freedom, prevention, access, and education. Such notions are mainly conceived for new tools (telemedicine, smartphone applications, home robots, etc.). However, when it comes to databases value is more difficult to evaluate (change of organization, risk assessment, evaluation of real-life practices and products, recognition of rare events by the exhaustiveness of situations, etc.). Artificial intelligence, which feeds on data, can be financed by the sale of its algorithms.

This begs a number of questions: Who do the data belong to? Can we talk about ownership (public or private) of data or should it be custody? Countries come up with different answers. Some allow data to be sold to merchants, others reserve them for research, yet others grant a monopoly (collection, analysis, applications) to public authorities. Patients creating the data are increasingly making their voices heard in this conductorless concert.

# What Data?

The question as to how to collect data from various sources rarely finds a consensual answer. Medical records are most often textual, paper based, and standardized. They must be transcribed to be the basis of digitized data, which means that language, syntax, and lexicons must be considered. The first decision nations need to make is whether to have electronic medical records from the outset either because the state is instituting the whole thing digitally (Estonia) or because the state wants to move to digital records for all in all sectors of care (the United States, Sweden).

The second decision nations need to make is whether to set up a centralized database (countries that have undergone a digital revolution in health) or to leave the dispersion of data to databases and connect them to a network to better preserve confidentiality and the risk for reidentification (as in France). Confidentiality is often used as a pretext for keeping data in the hands of "owners" and managing requests according to research "alliances." While the dispersion of data allows researchers to make choices and focus on the most reliable databases, their collection work is made more difficult and linking various sources on the same patient is complex (especially, if there are no common models or standards—medical records vary according to the care sector). As a result, databases built for a specific purpose are more efficient than general databases that are only used for specific research (genome banks, biological banks, imaging banks, etc.). In the United States health data of all kinds from more than 2000 sources are interrelated but not connected such as health data from the Department of Health and Human Service (HHS).

The major health databases are national (Denmark, Estonia) or regional (Basque Country, Catalonia).

Denmark was one of the first countries to gather all health data on a citizen in the same medical file. Moreover, each citizen is given a number from birth that is used for any function in society thus making multiple links possible. The medical file aggregates episodes of care including additional city and hospital examinations. It is secure. Patients can have access to their own information at any time via their medical files (sundhed.dk portal) and can grant permission to health professionals working with them to increment such information.

Other databases have been set up by insurers such as health maintenance organizations (HMOs) in the United States. Some insurance policies cover the entire country such as Medicare and Medicaid in the United States, CNAM (SNIIRAM) in France, or a large part of the country's population such as Clalit in Israel.

For example, Clalit in Israel is an insurance policy that covers half the population and includes everything under the same roof: city, hospital, home, telemedicine, etc. This allows there to be a permanent loop between needs and the implementation and evaluation of new means. The transfer of data in perspectives in new models is supported by strong research within the insurance company. Very positive results have been obtained in the management of renal failure, hospital readmissions, and personalization of high blood pressure treatment.

Hospitals are getting together to set up combined databases for clinical research. This is the case with major academic hospitals such as Imperial College, Oxford, Cambridge, University College London, Guy's, and St. Thomas's in the United Kingdom. A consortium of major integrated European cancer centers have pooled their data in the same format (Cancer Core Europe) and set up a federation of six European comprehensive cancer centers comprising DKFZ (Heidelberg), Cambridge Cancer Center, Val d'Hebron (Barcelona), NKI (Amsterdam), Karolinska Institute (Stockholm), and Gustave Roussy (Paris–Villejuif).

Hospital data warehouses are being set up by the same institution such as the Administration of Paris Public Hospitals (AP-HP). Some hospitals have gone so far as to create links between their data warehouses and large GAFA databases such as Google Deep Mind with the London Royal Free Hospital, which has led to population reactivation. Explorys is a very large clinical database set up by the Cleveland Clinic. It expanded and was acquired by IBM (Watson).[2]

Patients create commercial platforms such as Patients Know Best (a global organization) for their own data to give them some control over searches of their medical records. Some disease-specific databases are built by patient associations such as the European Multiple Sclerosis Data Alliance (MSDA) with sponsorship from the European Medicine Agency (EMA). The EMA encourages the creation of these registries by patient associations by setting up the Patient Registry Initiative. Some countries like Switzerland assert that healthcare system data legally belong to the patient.

Finally, there are private companies such as 23andMe that collect data. It currently sells genomic tests to increase data on susceptibility to diseases and has already acquired results covering more than 1 million people. It resells its data to pharmaceutical companies at prices that research teams cannot afford.

Data should always be available for research purposes and never denied. A case in point of the latter is the story of the African Ebola epidemic in 2014 where data could not be used even for research purposes because they had been collected by private telecommunications firms. This refusal provoked a violent reaction from the global scientific community and public health officials. Attempts are being made to reach an international agreement to allow free access to data (particularly, during epidemics) regardless of the public or private origin of the database.

## Which Sources for What Purposes?

Health data are usually gathered from medical files. It is easier to build databases from numerical data than from written data. In the United States the Information Technology Act (HITECH 2009) allows the Office of the National Coordinator for Health Information Technology (ONC) to issue certificates according to standards.

---

[2]https://www.technologyreview.com/s/536751/meet-the-health-care-company-ibm-needed-to-make-watson-more-insightful/.

In 2017 80% of physicians' records and 100% of hospital records were digitized facilitating the exchange of information as a result of these digitized files termed electronic health records (EHRs).[3]

Some countries such as Denmark, Estonia, and Hungary and health insurance companies such as Kaiser Permanente in the United States and Clalit in Israel collect, integrate, and structure health data with the aim of using them to improve the way care is provided, change practices, and facilitate disease prevention.

Other countries use different data collected for other purposes. For example, France makes use of reimbursement files through National Information System Inter Plans Health Insurance (SNIIRAM), hospital activity payment files through the Medicalization of In-training System Program (PMSI), and other sources. This requires linking all available data for each patient, deducing diagnoses from sources, and putting in place a useful basis for health policy research. The French database comprising 60 million people is much larger than that in other countries. Although available for research purposes since 2016, it can only be used for other purposes after recomposition, which requires several years of effort by teams of experts. In similar vein the National Patient-centered Clinical Research Network (PCORnet) set up by the Patient-centered Outcome Research Institute (PICORI) in the United States at a cost of USD250 million provides data for research.[4]

While most files in the French system were initially set up for payment purposes such as reimbursement, professional pay, and accounting, the databases are now used for research to improve practices in healthcare and epidemiology. This shift has been driven by change in the way care is provided, which is now patient centered and takes into account care provided by the city administration, hospitals, follow-up care, home and social care, as well as outcomes evaluated (not processes or the amount of care). This way of working allows health data on a large number of people to be used to refine decisions. Developing countries such as Estonia and Hungary have adopted such an all-digital system. Denmark is now at the forefront of such systems due to providing its citizens with unique citizen numbers. Insurance companies such as Medicare or Kaiser Permanente (United States) and Clalit (Israel) that coordinate all manner of activities have been able to include medical details and use them in their daily activities. As a result of the fragmented way data are collected in France— separately by the city administration, hospitals, and the social sector—coupled with the collection of data with the sole purpose of financial reimbursement and not of collecting vital details like diagnosis means that it is more or less impossible to have tools that can be easily used. This is why some databases such as the French National Institute of Health (INSERM) database are being built separately with "Sentinel" general practitioners for epidemiology or private initiatives focusing, in particular, on the consumption of drugs.

Wonders Info Co. (a.k.a. Wan Da Fullway Healthcare) is a private Chinese company that started operations in 2006 by providing a regional platform for the exchange

---

[3] Washington V., De Salvo K., Mostashari F., Blumenthal D., "The HITECH era and the path forward," *N Engl J Med*, 2017, 377, 10, 904–905.

[4] http://www.pcornet.org.

of health data in Shanghai. It currently covers 500 million people, 16 provinces, and 50 cities including Shanghai, Canton, Wuhan, Chengdu, and Xian. It is launching this year into deep learning and artificial intelligence to refine precision medicine using health parameters, personal data, and other data outside treatment.

Some countries have more recently embarked on constructing health databases specifically for research. The German Ministry of Research invested EUR150 million in 2017 to create a database using data from 17 hospitals and 40 partners. The European Medical Information Framework[5] is a recent European initiative to set up a health data platform for research.

Work on very specific research topics requires comprehensive databases (cohorts), databases including large numbers of cases (with the objective of improving epidemiology), or registers for medical devices and rare disease data. Each country has its own policy for these problems. International cooperation would be more effective and would save time and adopting the Scientific Panel for Health (SPH) proposal to create a European Research Institute for Health would be an important step forward.

However, Big Data on large numbers such as the study of the tumor genome or the study of the genome of patient populations have been collected by international cooperation. For example, the Global Alliance for Genomics and Health is a network of 400 institutions. The Heidelberg Centre (German Cancer Research Center) groups and sequences the tumor genomes of various centers (managing 10 TB per day, as much as Twitter) and analyzes data for medical applications. Europe has set up the Elixir program to build the infrastructure necessary for the exchange of laboratory data including genome sequences.

As for the genome the current trend in research is to no longer group data together in a single site from various centers (too cumbersome for transfer) but to send a search algorithm (owned by the researcher) to the various databanks that apply it to their data. The algorithm then collects the returned results for analysis.

In light of all this it is preferable to build databases that are specifically intended as tools for health research rather than recovering existing data collected for other purposes. These databases should be organized in such a way as to make it possible for people to be tested and monitored over time by artificial intelligence projects (continuous learning, prognosis, vigilance, etc.), whether general (care, health, vigilance, epidemiology) or specific (genome, imaging), to improve medical practices, the provision of care, disease prevention, and public health.

---

[5]http://www.emif.eu/.

# Characteristics

## Unique Number

Countries are split between those having a unique health identity number assigned at birth such as Denmark and Estonia and those doing everything possible to prohibit files from being linked to respect personal freedom such as France where an independent authority controls this prohibition (CNIL—Commission Nationale de l'Informatique et des Libertés). The OECD has identified 19 countries that have a unique citizen health identification number making it possible for all kinds of linkages between health and social sectors.[6]

Creating a database based on individuals having a unique number where all events in which the number is used aggregate is easier to operate than posing bans, obtaining authorizations, and going through successive controls to create links. However, this facility is at the cost of more fragile respect for privacy and the freedom of individuals. However, means of encrypting and restricting the reading of personal data to those authorized by the data subject (consent for a defined purpose) limit the risks for intrusion into private lives. The European directive on large databases requires privacy and accountability (i.e., to preserve the confidentiality of private data and to report on extractions and abuses). It is up to each country to make its own regulations based on these principles.

## Privacy: Anonymization and Consent

Personal data at the time information is entered and when they need to be linked with data of other files are recognizable whether pseudoanonymized (modifying the identity number according to a general rule) or not. However, anonymization does not ensure total confidentiality since there are means of finding the person as soon as linking brings in the many parameters needed for follow-up of health episodes over time.

Those hosting digitized data are more or less strictly regulated depending on the country when it comes to retrieving the file in the event of medical necessity.

There is a balance to be struck between respect for confidentiality and the research project. Public trust is central to the sustainability of databases. Some countries such as France favor privacy, while others such as Scotland leave it to a platform to judge the degree of anonymization to facilitate research. Scottish Informatics and Linkage Collaboration combines health and social field data for research.[7]

---

[6]Organisation for Economic Co-operation and Development, *Health Data Governance: Privacy, Monitoring and Research—Policy Brief* (Paris, France, OECD Publishing, October 2015): https://www.oecd.org/health/health-systems/Health-Data-Governance-Policy-Brief.pdfw.

[7]SILC Partners, Scottish Informatics and Linkage Collaboration: http://www.datalinkagescotland.co.uk/partners.

Scotland's Community Health Index registers people by providing them with a 10-digit number for clinical, public health, and other research purposes and to associate other files with the number.[8]

Scotland's Community Health Index was only initiated after public consultation to ensure public acceptance. It is maintained by an independent institution that has the right if necessary to conduct analyses on pseudoanonymized data. Personal data cannot be extracted from the secure warehouse. The balance between confidentiality and needs for each study is assessed pragmatically by adjusting the degree of anonymization to the risk level of data links.

The public's trust or, arguably more important, mistrust of these health databases strengthens or threatens their survival, respectively. Public consultation as happened in Scotland made it possible to go farther than usual in allowing analyses of personal data, even though it meant violating prohibitions. This can only happen if it comes from the population independent of any relationship with financiers, insurers, politicians, and other interested parties. If trust is lost, then everything is lost. It takes decades to regain trust.

An example of this occurred in England when the "care data" program ended dramatically. In the mistaken belief that the population would understand the value of the Health and Social Care Information Center (HSCIC) database based on the records of general practitioners (who are civil servants in this country) and hospitals, politicians in 2013 decided to create a database that culminated in a violent reaction from citizens. Citizens then demanded the right to privacy security and participation in any initiative based on their data. This very costly failure must make politicians think twice about trust and consent. The sensitive subject of social and health data requires not only consent but also the appropriation of such databases by the population.

Patient consent is a requirement for trust. When to ask for it? Is it necessary to be specific about the research done? Can presumed consent (which does not specify consent) be assumed? This sensitive subject of patient consent deserves special attention by all governments.

One way to maintain trust currently considered in the United States is to use block chains with closed and signed blocks. Each entry is made separately as a block. The blocks are linked with an encrypted signature. The chain increases with the number of entries and only partners in the chain can enter entries. The registration and signature of the author and verification of the data provide confidence to the patient and researcher while protecting privacy.[9] The Chinese company Wonders Info Co. (a.k.a. Wan Da Fullway Healthcare) is implementing block chains in its system this year.

---

[8]*Linking and Using Health and Social Care Data in Scotland: Charting a Way Forward*, report of meeting held May 22, 2014, Ninth, Edinburgh BioQuarter: http://www.scphrp.ac.uk/wp-content/uploads/2014/08/Health-and-Social-care-data-meeting-22-05-14-report.pdf.

[9]Redman J., "U.S. Gov't Announces Blockchain Healthcare Contest," Bitcoin.com: https://news.bitcoin.com/us-government-blockchain-healthcare/.

Estonia, which has a fully digitized system, is currently instituting medical record block chains to track any changes or additions whether voluntary or incongruous in real time. This would provide sufficient confidence to mix several sensitive sources and broaden the scope of research for improving care, the health system, and the environment of the population.

## Interoperability, Analysis, and Impact

### *Reliability*

The more complete, standardized, digitized, and designed the purpose for which data are collected (mainly medical records), the more reliable the analysis will be. This seems obvious, but few countries have managed to do so. Estonia has implemented such a plan; the United States and Sweden have been working toward it for more than 10 years; and France does not yet have a national system in which medical records are kept—even if it did it would not be standardized or digitized. The only source of medical records in France is the health insurance company that registers all prescriptions from city doctors. The company was set up solely for the purposes of reimbursement and hence does not record diagnoses, clinical histories, risk factors, or socioeconomic data. Connections between databases become ever-more problematic when they are not digitized. Can having many databases compensate for transcriptional errors and inaccuracies?

Germany through its Medical Informatics Initiative aims to improve care by facilitating exchanges between consortia made up of hospitals and city administrations and by using the national health database for research.

Developments in the way patient-centered care and the care pathway are provided, evaluating patient-reported outcome measures (PROMs) instead of processes and volumes of activity, requires that estimates from databases must be refined. Centers for Medicare and Medicaid Services (CMS) in the United States moved from fee-for-service to pay-per-episode (hospital and city administrations) in January 2015. This change is the result of setting up an accountable care organization (ACO) integrating city doctors and hospitals into the care pathway and requiring the digitization of pathway elements.

Clalit in Israel predicts real-life effects estimated from data considered reliable to customize treatments.

## The Use of Databases

The major problem with all these databases is their interoperability. This book demonstrates the analytical possibilities for epidemiology, disease prevention, and public health by providing many successful examples.

Technology assessment using databases could replace clinical trials in which patients are selected and followed for a limited period of time. This is all the more true when it comes to estimating the long-term risks posed by a product, the evaluation of treatments for chronic diseases, and the recognition of weak signals. Pharmacovigilance and material vigilance over decades will be possible. In France a study on the adverse effects of long-term diabetes drugs is in progress; it was brought about by reusing joint databases. The great advantage is the possibility of evaluating products for both efficacy and safety in real life including such factors as age, comorbidity, and polypharmacy. Authorities and agencies using such large databases can evaluate technologies in the knowledge they can make a real, independent assessment with no selection bias. No longer will comparisons be sought between two technologies, but between one or the other on large populations or subpopulations over several years. This will require standards used for technology assessment to be reformed.

Exploitation based on Big Data is currently specific to each research center where the main attraction is to discover unknown correlations (a.k.a. data mining). This is particularly the case in genomics and proteomics, which will be the source of new research. Epidemiology and disease prevention are also fields of exploration. All countries with such digitized databases are embarking on public health research in the national context.

As a result of data exploitation new ventures have been set up in which progressive learning takes place through an algorithm (author's property) and repetitions of an experience. Progress in this area is already effective (particularly, in imaging). The "intelligent" machine in imaging can replace the professional and the expert when it comes to reading an image. Moreover, its performance increases with the degree of learning (radiology, Cardiologs ECG Analysis Solution, pathology, etc.). Algorithms do a better job than an on-call resident at detecting pulmonary embolisms. Soon many diagnoses will be automatically made from parameter surveys and images.[10]

Wherever in the world artificial intelligence has brought about a breakthrough that helps medical practice it then spreads throughout the world. There is therefore no national particularity apart from the incentive to create new companies (financial incentive) or for a public research institution to develop an algorithm open to all (international recognition). From study of the environment to smart cities, pollution, etc., through to the prevention of rat infestations—all demonstrate the extent to which the field of health has expanded across all fields or, conversely, the interest shown in considering health as an important part of any new program of society made possible by the availability of databases. China has major projects for new cities built on

---

[10]Kligerman S.J., Lahiji K., Galvin J.R., Stokum C., White C.S., "Missed Pulmonary Emboli on CT Angiography: Assessment with Pulmonary Embolism Computer-Aided Detection," *American Journal of Roentgenology*, 2014, 202(1), 65–73.

exploiting multiple learning (meteorology, transport, pollution, etc.) that will have a positive impact on the health of citizens.

A new industry (i.e., artificial intelligence) in the field of health along with the emergence of new companies that are taking or will take a global place are paving the way for a new economy.

# Control

Faced with the proliferation of applications the future will shortly bring, it seems essential to standardize databases to safeguard privacy and make database "owners" responsible. The legislator has a duty to delimit the ways in which personal data are shared and any possible links to such data. It will be the population who determine the degree of prohibition in inverse proportion to the possibilities of exploitation. The balance between limits on use and incentives for innovation and between restriction and the creation of new companies is delicate.

In any event such databases must be protected. The European General Data Protection Regulations that came into force on May 25, 2018 aim to protect individuals.

Any administrative complication, even with the good intention to protect the citizen, will further hinder the implementation of data collection in Europe.

In a judgment of December 7, 2017 the European Court of Justice concluded: "Software, one of the functionalities of which allows the use of patient-specific data, in particular for the purpose of detecting contraindications, drug interactions and excessive dosages, constitutes, with respect to that functionality, a medical device within the meaning of those provisions, even if such software does not act directly in or on the human body." This decision does not apply to applications of *quantified* welfare *self*. The court issued a reading grid making it possible to determine products that not only must be certified in France by an approved institution, but also in accordance with the rules of the High Authority for Health (HAS) and of course the CE[11] marking.

The CE marking coupled now with registering software as devices in Title II or Title III represents a double penalty suggesting a mountain of paperwork to be completed and a maze of administrative offices to be contacted. Where are the data warehouses, analysis software, and algorithms whose purposes are to improve care and detect contraindications and interactions? It could be argued that anonymization makes the term "patient-specific" redundant, although the text specifies that this applies to the "exploitation" of patient data (including collection, which is the case in the construction of Big Data) and not restricted to care assistance for the patient (improving personal medical outcome). Legal battles can be seen in the offing!

Data piracy is of great concern to citizens. Millions of digitized medical records are reported to have been hacked. A ransom was demanded from the Hollywood

---

[11] *Legalis*, January 12, 2018.

Presbyterian Medical Center in 2016. Massachusetts General Hospital and Kansas Heart Hospital were also reportedly victims of piracy. Currently, digital surveillance services report that the health sector is the main target of piracy. The more data (especially, hospital care data) are digitized, the greater the risk. Moreover, preventing this risk is not a question of money but of skills, contrary to what is generally believed.

Cybersecurity therefore takes precedence when building a health database. Hospitals that do not have the same resources as those of public or private giants are the most vulnerable (especially, since they have a large cash flow at their disposal). The fable of the wolf and the lambs is still in the news.

## Conclusion

Database architecture when adapted to a search facilitates exploitation irrespective of whether it involves the analysis or construction of algebraic algorithms of artificial intelligence. Providing citizens with unique identification numbers, as happens in Denmark, makes it possible to use databases from a variety of sources; otherwise, linking requires interoperability between databases. The degree of anonymization at the time of data collection varies according to the citizen's desire for privacy protection and the need for linking between various different databases.

Public acceptance of the use of personal databases is based on trust. Trust is fragile as revealed by delayed collective reactions in England. Transparency, independent governance of funders (insurers) and regulators (health leaders and organizers), and ownership of the foundations by citizens themselves help to build trust. Facebook revealed in March 2018 that it had transmitted the data of 50 million people for electoral purposes. In so doing it demonstrated just how quickly people's confidence in such databases can be lost.

Finally, the risk of being held to ransom as a result of data piracy (particularly, within often very vulnerable health institutions) remains a topical issue that is difficult to circumvent. The use of block chains to increase trust and minimize risk is currently a path being followed by some countries such as Estonia, the United States, and China.

**Human**

# Are Public Health Issues Endangered by Information?

**Gérald Bronner**

Deregulation of the internet information market is one of the major technological developments of the new millennium. It would therefore be surprising if its contributions to our social life were perfectly unambiguous. This is particularly the case if attention is focused on health issues and how information is now being disseminated on the fundamental human concern of health. To what extent do patients use the internet to self-diagnose? To what extent do they consult the internet looking for a prediagnosis before going to see the doctor? How can public opinion movements influence certain political decisions or collective norms that do not always agree with what methodical rationality might prescribe or even with certain legal decisions? These are some of the urgent questions that arise today.

The internet is a formidable provider of information making specialized data that were previously beyond the reach of ordinary citizens available to them (especially, those who did not frequent the social environments in which such data were produced). The internet is also a tool that allows for many resources to be pooled. A good example is Foldit, a game that allows internet users to freely try molecular combinations to better understand how proteins can be deployed in space. The game has led to the publication of three articles, one in the highly prestigious journal *Nature*. Such mutualization also makes it possible to break free from "spatial" limits of research. Since scientists cannot be everywhere when it comes to classifying and identifying rare phenomena it makes very good sense to make use of the many. A good example is the Tela Botanica network that connects tens of thousands of botanists—some professional, some amateur—to effectively review France's entire plant nomenclature. Pooling of resources can be particularly useful when it comes to identifying rare disease symptoms that at times are considered little more than statistical anomalies. It is said that research into muscular dystrophy has benefited

G. Bronner (✉)
Académie des Technologies, Académie Nationale de Médecine, University of Paris, Paris, France
e-mail: gerald.bronner@univ-paris-diderot.fr

© Springer Nature Switzerland AG 2020
B. Nordlinger et al. (eds.), *Healthcare and Artificial Intelligence*,
https://doi.org/10.1007/978-3-030-32161-1_31

from the effects of data sharing.[1] The availability of such information may have many virtues, but I will focus here on reasons causing concern. Despite the huge progress made in information availability, a number of beliefs persist and even have developed that contradict scientific knowledge among which mistrust of vaccines is causing a lot of worry. Indeed, a vast comparative survey covering 67 countries showed how widespread these beliefs had become and that France was one of the worst affected in this regard. Another survey pointed out that 38.2% of French people were against vaccination in 2013, whereas this percentage in 2000 was much lower at 8.5%.[2,3,4]

Mistrust regarding vaccines has become emblematic of questions we ask ourselves about the internet. Should the fundamental problem of deregulating the information market be reformulated? It is not so much the availability of information that we must question, but its visibility. I will deal with the problem by looking at it from three different angles within the volumetric limits of this text.

## Minority Tyranny

The internet creates fewer new phenomena than it amplifies old ones. Thus, many commentators have argued that social life tends to place the majority of individuals including those in democracies under the supervision of active minorities. Moreover, several studies from what is known as the "new science of networks"[5] or "web science"[6] clearly show that this phenomenon has amplified. By assembling a number of very important databases such studies reveal that a small number of motivated people can influence opinion on the internet much more than in traditional social life.[7] With reference to theses of the Columbia School such motivated people are termed "super opinion leaders" (Gladwell 2002). While some authors see in the internet the hope of democratizing democracy, all these studies show that the democracy in question does not necessarily correspond to the ideal they seem to be worried about: some vote a thousand times, while others never do.[8] However, motivated

[1]Callon M., Lascoumes P., Barthe Y., *Acting in an uncertain world. Essai sur la démocratie technique*, Paris, Le Seuil, 2001, p. 77.

[2]https://www.ebiomedicine.com/article/S2352-3964(16)30398-X/fulltext.

[3]Peretti-Watel P., Verger P., Raude J., Constant A., Gautier A., Jestin C., Beck F., "Dramatic change in public attitudes towards vaccination…," *Euro Surveill*, 2013, 18, 44.

[4]What Robert Michels called "the bronze law of oligarchy." Michels R., *Les Partis politiques, Essai sur les tendances oligarchiques des démocraties*, Paris, Flammarion, 1971.

[5]Watts D.J., "The "new" science of networks," *Annual Review of Sociology*, 2004, 30, 243–270.

[6]Hendler J., Hall W., Shadbolt N., Berners-Lee T., Weitzner D., "Web science: An interdisciplinary approach to understanding the Web," *Web Science*, 2008, 51, 7, 60–69.

[7]Watts D.J., Strogatz S., "Collective dynamics of "Small-World" Networks," *Nature*, 1998, 393, 6684, 440–442.

[8]Cardon D., *La démocratie Internet*, Paris, Seuil, 2010; Leadbeater C., Miller P., *The Pro-Am Revolution: How Enthusiasts Are Changing Our Economy and Society*, London, Demos, 2004; Flichy P., *Le sacre de l'amateur*, Paris, Seuil, 2010.

believers such as antivaccination activists "vote" a lot.[9] This is shown by a recent study of the activity of some antivaccine internet users on social networks, which has all the reticular characteristics of what web science literature pointed out under the term "small world." These small worlds have two characteristics according to Shirky.[10] The first is that "small groups of network nodes" are strongly interconnected allowing them to better disseminate their views than "large groups of nodes" whose networks are weakly interconnected. The second characteristic is that they are more robust and resistant to damage than these large groups. Therefore, by randomly removing through a mind experiment the nodes of this type of network no significant impact on the efficiency and dynamics of information flow will be observed. The immediate effect of this activity when it comes to religious minorities (particularly, in the field of health) is to bring about permanent confusion between the visibility of information on a deregulated cognitive market and its representativeness. This asymmetry of motivation is crucial to understanding how credulity spreads.[11] Walter Quatrociocchi and his team[12] were able to show recently that on the Italian Facebook network, for example, there was three times more conspiracy content sharing than scientific content. Thus, many of our fellow citizens who are undecided on technical issues such as adjuvants for vaccines may be impressed by the salience of certain intellectual proposals that, if not opposed with robust arguments, will spread easily allowing ideas that were previously confined to the margins of radicalism to spread in the public space.

## Cognitive Demagogy

There is a second fundamental point that makes it possible to understand why the new structure of the cognitive market favors sometimes irrational relationships to public health issues. This is part of what can be called cognitive demagogy. It happens that some misconceptions dominate, persist, and sometimes have more success than more reasonable and balanced ideas because they capitalize on questionable intellectual processes that are attractive to the mind. A recent study has shown that misinformation spreads on average six times faster than more demanding information[13] and another study points out that it is better memorized.[14] A possible explanation for such a phenomenon (i.e., the virality of the false) is that it flatters the most intuitive but

---

[9]Watts D.J., Strogatz S., op. cit.

[10]Shirky C., *Here Comes Everybody: The Power of Organizing without Organizations*, New York, Penguin Press, 2008.

[11]For more on this point see Bronner G., *La démocratie des crédules*, Paris, Puf, 2013.

[12]Bessi A., Zollo F., Del Vicario M., Scala, A. Cardarelli G., Quattrociocchi W., "Trend of Narratives in the Age of Misinformation," arXiv, 2015, 1504.05163v1.

[13]Vosoughi S., Roy D., Aral S., "The spread of true and false news online," *Science*, 2018, 359, 6380, 1146–1151.

[14]Pantazi M., Kissine M., Klein O., "The power of the truth bias: False information affects memory and judgment even in the absence of distraction," *Social Cognition* (to appear).

not always the most honorable inclinations of our mind. Our brain, for example, has an appetite for zero risk, focuses its attention on the costs rather than the benefits of a proposal, and more easily takes into account the consequences of its action rather than its inaction. All these banal elements of our psychological life have been experimentally tested, often replicated, and make it possible to understand why ceteris paribus some alarmist proposals in terms of public health will be more successful than more reasonable approaches.[15] Perhaps these mental dispositions were once useful in a particularly threatening environment, but at a time when threats are much more controlled by the dominant species we have become and when at the same time information that claims to alert us to a danger is produced in industrial quantities we are likely to be confronted with a form of long-term precautionary ideology called precautionism.[16]

## Poisoned Beliefs

Precautionary narratives that spread are often inconsistent. In 2009 some residents of the city of St. Cloud in Minnesota began to experience curious symptoms: headaches, nasal discomfort, strange sensations such as having a metallic taste in the mouth. The residents came to understand that the cause of these adverse effect was the recent installation of three relay stations. The case seemed all the more serious to them because they had been installed not far from a retirement home and a nursery school. The collective made up of concerned individuals that alerted the entire city planned to file a complaint and soon the media intervened to denounce this health scandal and the plight of those living near the city who were trying unsuccessfully to find ways of filtering out the waves from the relay stations. After the case had made a lot of noise, it was realized that the signal-processing electronic bays had not yet been installed and that connection to the electricity grid had not yet taken place. In short, these antennas were inactive and did not emit any waves! What had happened in St. Cloud was an epidemic of sincerely felt symptoms. This does not mean that individuals were not really suffering since they were suffering from having believed alarmist stories rather than the effect of the non-existent waves. However psychosomatic such suffering may be, it is still very real. Indeed, as shown in a study conducted by neuroscientists[17] using functional magnetic resonance imaging (fMRI), people who declare themselves sensitive to waves react significantly more than others to fictitious exposure by a specific modification of the activity of the anterior cingulate cortex and the island cortex. In other words, endorsing the story of hypersensitivity to the presence of waves stimulates what experts call a "pain neuromatrix." Similarly,

---

[15]Kahneman D., *System 1 System 2. Les deux vitesses de la pensée*, Paris, Flammarion, 2012.

[16]Bronner G., Géhin E., *L'inquiétant principe de précaution*, Paris, Puf, 2010.

[17]Landgrebe M., Barta W., Rosengarth K., Frick U., Hauser S., Langguth B., Rutschmann R., Greenlee M.W., Hajak G., Eichhammer P., "Neuronal correlates of symptom formation in functional somatic syndromes: An fMRI study," *Neuroimage*, July 2008, 41(4), 1336–1344.

psychologists[18] have shown that being exposed to a television report on the harmful effects of electromagnetic fields on health not only causes a feeling of anxiety but also an increase in the reported perception of fictitious Wi-Fi stimulation! Anxiety stories that spread are not always without effect. The expression "prevention is better than cure" is here not as wise as it might seem. Indeed, prevention can sometimes make you sick or rather make you feel sick. Alarms on public health topics are sometimes useful, but at other times they can inconsistently contribute to an epidemic of misperceived symptoms. Moreover, this was shown in another way by a study[19] undertaken by researchers from the Sydney School of Public Health indicating a link between the spatial and temporal distribution of health complaints and the activity of opposition groups in these fields. Such complaints contribute to the dissemination of narrative proposals that promote the nocebo effect. Some alerts can therefore be poisoned to some extent because they are not without consequences at least with regard to the criterion of well-being that the WHO now includes in its very definition of health status. They create a "bottleneck" of fears because denying them takes time (especially, when it comes to health issues): the time of science is not the unbridled time of the information market. Some individuals genuinely suffer, but perhaps not because of the cause they imagine. They are suffering from beliefs.

## Some Tracks

A common mistake here is to believe that nothing need be done to preserve individual freedoms (particularly, that of free speech). The opposite is true. Inaction in this area is one way of entrenching the domination of cognitive demagogy. There are many ways to find solutions to this considerable problem, but I will only mention two that directly involve the possible mobilization of artificial intelligence. The first is what is called the architecture of choice or nudge.[20] Since a major problem with the current cognitive market is, if we spin the metaphor, the way in which the shelves are crowded, especially the heads of gondolas". Clearly, the way an intellectual proposal on a particular subject is endorsed (especially, if we are undecided about it) will be statistically impacted by the way in which argumentative visibility is organized. Algorithms that give prominence to some intellectual proposals over others need to be thoroughly rethought. It is a question of implementing normative devices (morality, in a way) because these algorithms are certainly not neutral, but the consequence of their activity is still incompletely thought out. Such devices would not be liberticidal

---

[18]Bräscher A.K., Raymaekers K., Van den Bergh O., Witthöft M., "Are media reports able to cause somatic symptoms attributed to WiFi radiation? An experimental test of the negative expectation hypothesis," *Environmental Research*, July 2017, 156, 265–271.

[19]Chapman S., St George A., Waller K., Cakic V., "The pattern of complaints about Australian wind farms does not match the establishment and distribution of turbines: Support for the psychogenic, 'communicated disease' hypothesis," *PLoS One*, 2013, 8:e76584.

[20]Thaler R.H., Sunstein Q.C., *Nudge. La méthode douce pour inspirer la bonne décision*, Paris, Vuibert, 2010.

because it is not a question of censoring content but of thinking about the conditions that prevail in the cognitive market and taking into account considerations relating to general interest (in particular, in the field of health). Put concretely, is it acceptable to have a situation in which searches for all kinds of subjects depend on the order of appearance and the number of proposals based on belief rather than science using a search engine like Google? Is it possible to extract the cognitive market from the tyranny of minorities?

Another way to use artificial intelligence here is to view it as a cognitive prosthesis that if properly deployed can remove certain misconceptions that weigh so heavily and endemically on our judgment. When it comes to other subjects artificial intelligence seems to be able to be set up in a satisfactory way. For instance, the human brain, even a well-meaning one, will have the greatest difficulty in freeing itself from stereotypes that will force it to make decisions that are not always reasonable. Evidence shows that certain ethnic groups suffer handicaps when it comes to recruitment or leasing. Could machines help us to reduce the share of injustice in some of our decisions? The use of artificial intelligence in professional recruitment is already commonplace. Since the turn of the century 95% of large companies and more than half of SMEs have been using an automated CV processing system called the Applicant Tracking System that identifies desired keywords by job type. Over the past 10 months, a large-scale experiment has been conducted in the United States by Unilever, a giant of the American economy. This involves selecting applicants by means of cognitive assessment based on the artificial intelligence of the Pymetric platform, then giving them a video interview, and finally subjecting the interview to analysis by the HireVue program. The results reported by Unilever over a recruitment year are more than interesting. First, they show, unsurprisingly, that response times are drastically reduced from four months to four weeks. They then indicate that the acceptance rate of candidates increases from 62 to 82% proving that the procedure makes it easier for the offer to meet demand on the labor market. Finally, they show that the machine, less subject to stereotypical effects, tends to introduce much more diversity into its proposals than would a human brain. Thus, universality represented in the recruitment phase increased from 840 to 2600 and the number of non-white candidates increased significantly. Provided that algorithms are indexed to universalist values, artificial intelligence in many fields could free us from some of our cultural assumptions and better open our minds to possibilities. Clearly, if such cognitive prostheses succeed in reducing the weight of stereotypes, they could also limit the influence of cognitive demagogy, but in a way that has yet to be invented.

# Social and Emotional Robots: Useful Artificial Intelligence in the Absence of Consciousness

Laurence Devillers

## Realities and Fantasies

Artificial intelligence and robotics are opening up important opportunities in the field of health diagnosis and treatment support with aims like better patient follow-up. A social and emotional robot is an artificially intelligent machine that owes its existence to computer models designed by humans. If it has been programmed to engage in dialogue, detect and recognize emotional and conversational cues, adapt to humans, or even simulate humor, such a machine may on the surface seem friendly. However, such emotional simulation must not hide the fact that the machine has no consciousness.

However, it should not be forgotten that artificial intelligence and robotics are little more than fantasies. In 2016 AlphaGo (an artificial intelligence computer program designed by Google DeepMind) succeeded in beating Lee Sedol, one of the best go players. The victory raised questions about the promise held by and risks for using intelligent machines. However, although this feat, much like Deep Blue's victory over chess champion Garry Kasparov some 20 years ago, may well lead us to fantasize about what robots will be capable of tomorrow in our daily lives, it should not. When AlphaGo beats a go player the machine is unaware of what it's doing. The robot can succeed in a difficult task and will not brag about it unless it has been programmed to simulate an emotional state. The robot is a complex object capable of simulating cognitive abilities but in the absence of human consciousness, feelings, or that desire or "appetite for life" that Spinoza refers to as *conatus*[1] (effort to persevere in being) which refers to everything from the mind to the body.

---

[1] *Ethics* III, prop. 9, *scolie* [grammatical remark].

---

L. Devillers (✉)
Artificial Intelligence and Ethics, Sorbonne-Université/LIMSI, CNRS, Orsay, France
e-mail: laurence.devillers@limsi.fr

B. Nordlinger et al. (eds.), *Healthcare and Artificial Intelligence*,
https://doi.org/10.1007/978-3-030-32161-1_32

Artificial intelligence is already being used to detect cancers; read emotions on a face; and imitate artists, painters, or musicians. Tests have proven the incredible capabilities of software such as Sony's Spotify Flow Machines. Improvisations incorporating Bach's style become indistinguishable from the original author, even for experts of the German composer. Although machines will be able to create by imitation or by chance, they will not be able to know if what they have created is interesting because they have no conscience. Human choice will always be essential.

Despite impressive performances on specific tasks, it should be kept in mind that artificial intelligence systems can only learn from "real data" and only use past data to predict the future. However, many of the discoveries of our greatest scientists are due to the ability to be counterintuitive—to ignore current knowledge! In the 16th century Galileo had the intuition that the weight of an object had no influence on the speed at which it falls. The law of physics that states "all bodies fall at the same speed in a void" cannot be inferred from observations of the real world. Serenity (a.k.a. the "gift of finding" at random) likewise is not the strength of the machine. Faced with a question without a known answer the human being is incredibly stronger than the machine at coming up with solutions. For the machine to integrate intentionality and human-like creativity seems very hard to imagine. So, isn't the term artificial intelligence for unconscious machines inappropriate? Nevertheless, all these so-called intelligence tools comprising "weak" artificial substances become formidable allies when part of complementary interaction with humans. Social and emotional robotics wants to create companion robots that will supposedly provide us with therapeutic assistance or even monitor such assistance. In the case of neurodegenerative pathologies or severe disabilities the robot may even be better than humans at interacting with people. The machine is in tune with other, very slow, almost inhuman rhythms. The robot listens in a non-critical way and impatiently. For very lonely people the machine can also avoid depressions that lead to dementia. It is necessary to learn how to use these new tools without fear and to understand their usefulness.

## Intelligence and Consciousness of Robots

Intelligence is often described as the ability to learn to adapt to the environment or to modify the environment to adapt it to the individual's own needs. A robot is a platform that embeds a large amount of computer software into various algorithmic approaches in perceptions of, decisions about, and actions in our environment. Even though every object perception module or face recognition module is driven by machine learning algorithms, automation of all modules is very complex to adjust. Reinforcement algorithms that require humans to design reward metrics are used to give the robot the ability to learn autonomously from its environment. The robot learns by trial and error according to programmed rewards in a clumsy and laborious way and combines actions in the world and internal representations to achieve the particular tasks for which it is designed.

Children learn by experiencing the world. Robots are called "intelligent" because they too can learn. Although such a task is extremely difficult for a robot because it has neither instinct nor intentions to make decisions, it can imitate the human being. Robots feel nothing and have no conscience despite the fact that they can be programmed to empathetically say "I feel sorry for you!" Machines will become increasingly autonomous, talkative, and emotionally gifted through sophisticated artificial intelligence programs, but they will not be capable of the feelings, creativity, and imagination that are understood as human. The machine cannot feel "sad" because it is devoid of consciousness of any phenomena. Moreover, it cannot "understand" the concept of sadness in the human sense.

At present any relative autonomy possessed by robots is still programmed by humans. Such programmed learning ability can offer varying degrees of freedom to the machine. Giving a robot the ability to learn alone, in interaction with the environment, or in interaction with humans is the Holy Grail of artificial intelligence researchers. It is therefore desirable to teach robots common and moral values of life in society. The ability to learn alone constitutes a technological and legal breakthrough and raises many ethical questions. Such robots can be creative and autonomous in their decision-making if and only if they are programmed for this.

Any attempt to copy the intelligence of humans to a machine is simply narcissistic because we know little about human intelligence. We do not understand the substratum of thought and are unaware that some of our organs act autonomously. We are only aware of what we can perceive and think about. There is no more polysemic and interpretable term than "consciousness." For some it refers to self-awareness; for others it refers to the consciousness of others, to phenomenal consciousness, to moral consciousness, etc.

As a result of the materialistic way life is conceived the computer and the human brain can be considered comparable systems capable of manipulating information. The most efficient numerical models such as deep learning are based on simplified modeling of the neuron (formerly, neurone) integrated in a discrete-state machine simulated on a computer. The number of hidden layers of the model architecture correspond to the depth. For the moment we are very far from understanding the complexity of life. Experiments conducted in the NeuroSpin project by Stanislas Dehaene's team (particularly, using subliminal images) have shown that our brain functions mainly in subconscious mode. Routine actions such as the recognition of faces and words are carried out without recourse to consciousness. The human brain sets up two types of information processing to access consciousness. The first type called "global availability" corresponds to the vast repertoire of information and modular programs that can be assembled at any time for their use. The second type corresponds to information processing that is specific to the human consciousness such as self-monitoring or self-evaluation (i.e., the ability to process information about oneself, a.k.a. "metacognition"). Thus, the brain is able to introspect, control its own process, and obtain information about itself—attributes that lead to autonomy.

Current artificial intelligence systems are capable of correlating facts with deep-learning approaches for such purposes as decision-making and learning without being aware of them. However, some robot prototypes already have embryos endowed with "consciousness" levels comparable with those described by Stanislas Dehaene. They have been simulated through knowledge sharing and introspection.

However, robots are not conscious the same way humans are. Robots do not possess moral or criminal consciousness nor do they experience qualitative consciousness such as feeling hot or cold and feeling anxious because they have no viscera. This will not change unless once again a way can be found to simulate them. Artificial consciousness endowed with feelings, thoughts, and free will without human programming is therefore unlikely to emerge spontaneously from current computer architectures.

## Social and Emotional Robotics in Health

What value do robots have when it comes to health? By 2060 it is expected that 32% of the French population will be over 60 years old, an increase of 80% in 50 years. Dependency and chronic diseases will go hand in hand with such aging. Robots can be very useful in following patients throughout an illness and helping sick, elderly, and/or disabled people to stay at home and reduce their periods of hospitalization. Robots are available 24/7, are patient, can overcome perceptual deficiencies (deafness, visual impairment), and provide access to information on the internet more easily than a computer. They are also valuable when it comes to continuously recording data and sending them to a doctor to detect abnormal behaviors (depression, stress, etc.) and to follow patients suffering from bipolar disorders, Holter disease, and degenerative diseases to ascertain their effects on daily life. It is already possible to design intelligent systems to train people suffering cognitive impairment to stimulate memory and language. Currently, although robots are not really autonomous and have no consciousness, no emotions, no desires like humans, human capacities are being projected on them. This is the reason it is essential not only to consider how to regulate the way they work, but also to demystify their capacities (in particular, through education), make them more transparent, and understand the computer programs they have on board.

## Emotional Interaction with Machines

Establishing an emotional interaction with robots is no longer science fiction but an emerging theme for[2] many research teams including that of the author. The domain is called affective computing.[3] At LIMSI-CNRS (Laboratoire d'informatique pour la mécanique et les sciences de l'ingénieur/Centre national de la recherche) we are

---

[2]Reeves B., Nass C., *The Media Equation: How People Treat Computers, Television, and New Media like Real People and Places*, Cambridge University Press, 1996.

[3]Picard R.W., *Affective Computing*, MIT Press, 1997.

working to give robots the ability to recognize emotions and be empathetic so that they can best help their users. We teach them to enter into dialogue and analyze emotions using verbal and non-verbal cues such as acoustic cues (e.g., laughter) to adapt their responses.[4]

Social robots will share our space, live in our homes, help us in our work and daily life, and share a certain story with us. Why not give them some machine humor? Humor plays a crucial role in social relationships: it dampens stress, builds confidence, and creates complicity between people. If you are alone and unhappy, the robot could crack a joke to comfort you; if you are angry, it could help you put things into perspective saying that the situation is not as bad as you think. It could also be self-deprecating if it makes mistakes and realizes it! How should such "empathetic" robots be welcomed? This can only be ascertained by conducting perceptual studies on human–machine interactions. LIMSI-CNRS has conducted numerous laboratory and EHPAD (Etablissement d'Hébergement pour Personnes Agées Dépendantes; nursing homes) tests with elderly people and in rehabilitation centers with the association Approche[5] as part of the BPI ROMEO2[6] project led by SoftBank Robotics.[7] Created in 1991 the main mission of the association Approche is to promote new technologies (robotics, electronics, home automation, information and communication technologies, etc.) for the benefit of people with disability regardless of age and living environment. We also conducted studies into everyday life activities such as games with Professor Anne-Sophie Rigaud's team at the Living Lab of Broca[8] Hospital. All these experiments have shown that robots are quite well accepted by patients when they have time to experiment with them. Postexperimental discussions also raised a number of legitimate concerns about the lack of transparency and explanations of the way in which such robots behave.

Developing an interdisciplinary research discipline involving computer scientists, doctors, and cognitive psychologists to study the effects of coevolution with these

---

[4]Devillers L., Tahon M., Sehili M., Delaborde A., "Detection of affective states in spoken interactions: Robustness of non-verbal cues," *TAL*, 2014, 55(2); "Inference of human beings' emotional states from speech in human–robot interactions," *International Journal of Social Robotics,* 2015, 7(4), 451–463.

[5]http://www.approche-asso.com.

[6]A first collaborative project, ROMEO funded by the FUI (Fonds Unique Interministériel), between 2009 and 2012, worked to specific the needs for a robot able to provide assistance to people in situations of loss of autonomy and to develop the prototype of a large humanoid robot. In 2013, the ROMEO2 project, within the framework of the PSPC (Structuring Project of the Competitiveness Poles) funded by Bpifrance, took over with the objective of evaluating, over the duration, the interest of a robot assistant in the domestic environment. This is a far-reaching project, and Softbank robotics has been working in coordination with more than a dozen academic and industrial partners, including LIMSI-CNRS on emotion detection in spoken interaction.

[7]Kumar Pandey A., Gelin R., Alami R., Vitry R., Buendia A., Meertens R., Chetouani M., Devillers L., Tahon M., Filliat D., Grenier Y., Maazaoui M., Kheddar A., Lerasle F., Fitte Duval L., "Ethical considerations and feedback from social human–robot interaction with elderly people," *AIC*, 2014.

[8]Garcia M., Bechade L., Dubuisson Duplessis G., Pittaro G., Devillers L., "Towards Metrics of Evaluation of Pepper Robot as a Social Companion for Elderly People," *International Workshop on Spoken Dialog System Technology 2017.*

machines over the long term is urgent. The machine will learn to adapt to us, but how will we adapt to it?

## Ethics of Robotic Systems

We must avoid not only a lack of trust but also too blind a trust in artificial intelligence programs. A number of ethical values are important such as the deontology and responsibility of designers; the emancipation of users, evaluation, transparency, explainability, loyalty, and equity of systems; and the study of human–machine coevolution.

Social and emotional robots raise many ethical, legal, and social issues. Who is responsible in case of an accident: the manufacturer, the buyer, the therapist, or the user? How should the way robots work be regulated? Should moral rules be included in their programming? Should their use be controlled through permits? For what tasks do we want to create these artificial entities? How should our privacy and personal data be preserved?

Any system must be evaluated before it is placed in the hands of users.[9] How should artificial intelligence that learns from and adapts to humans be evaluated? How should artificial intelligence that learns on its own be evaluated? Can it be proven that it will be limited to the functions for which it was designed and that it will not exceed the limits set? Who will oversee the data the machine selects for its learning and ensure the data are directed at certain actions?

These important issues have only recently been raised. The dramatic advances in digital technology will one day improve people's well-being provided we think about what we want to do with it—not about what we can do with it.

This is the reason the Institute of Electrical and Electronics Engineers (IEEE), the largest international professional digital association and a global scholarly organization, launched an initiative to get researchers to reflect on ethics related to self-designated systems.[10] As a result about a dozen working groups on norms and standards have emerged[11] including on robot nudging (incentive manipulation) for which the author of this chapter is responsible. CERNA[12] (Commission de réflexion sur

---

[9]Dubuisson Duplessis G., Devillers L., "Towards the consideration of dialogue activities in engagement measures for human–robot social interaction," *International Conference on Intelligent Robots and Systems, Designing and Evaluating Social Robots for Public Settings Workshop, 2015*, pp. 19–24.

[10]Standards.ieee.org/develop/industry-connections/ec/autonomoussystems.html.

[11]Fagella D., "IEEE Standards and Norms Initiative": techemergence.com/ethics-artificial-intelligence-business-leaders/.

[12]Allistene's Reflection Commission on Research Ethics in Digital Science and Technology: cerna-ethics-allistene.org.

l'Éthique de la Recherche en sciences et technologies du Numérique d'Allistene) also took up this subject.[13]

Artificial intelligence has the potential to provide better health diagnoses, stimulation tools, detection of abnormal behaviors, and better assistance (particularly, for disability or loss of autonomy). Although machines will be able to learn on their own, they will not be able to know whether what they have learned is interesting because they have no conscience. Human control will always be essential. It will also be necessary to develop ethical frameworks for social robots (particularly, in health) and to understand the level of human–machine complementarity.

In the author's book *Robots and Humans: Myths, Fantasies and Reality*[14] the author of this chapter proposes to enrich Asimov's laws with commands adapted to ensure robots assist in everyday life. The foundations of such "commandments" stem in part from feedback from interactions between elderly people and robots. The challenge is to formulate them in algorithmic form.

Some commands are generic to all numerical applications, while others are specific to the social robot:

1  Privacy: "You will not disclose my data to anyone."
2  Right to be forgotten: "You will forget everything I ask you to forget."
3  Security: "You will disconnect from the internet if I ask you to."
4  Control: "You will be regularly controlled to evaluate what you have learned."
5  Explainability and traceability: "You will explain your behavior to me if I ask you to."
6  Loyalty: "You will be loyal."
7  Consent: "You will be empathetic and simulate emotions only if I am aware of it!"
8  Risk of dependence: "You will stimulate my memory and make sure that I don't become too dependent on you!"
9  Danger of confusion: "You will be careful that I do not confuse you with a human being!"
10  Adapting to social rules: "You will learn to live with humans and adapt to social rules."
11  Utility and kindness: "You will be benevolent and useful and do so with a little humor!"

Despite the dearth of such "commandments, it is important to start building ethical and safe behaviors into the social robots of tomorrow. We need to demystify artificial intelligence, train the public in artificial intelligence, and put the values of human beings right at the center of the design of such robotic systems.

---

[13]Grinbaum A., Chatila R., Devillers L., Ganascia J.-G., Tessier C., Dauchet M., "Ethics in robotics research," *IEEE Robotics & Automation Magazine*, 2017, 24(3), 139–145.

[14]Devillers L., *Robots and Humans: Myths, Fantasies and Reality*, Plon, 2017.

# Augment Humans, and Then What?

Guy Vallancien

Relayed from network to network, bugled from media to media by preachers of revelation or paradise whose audience success swells with the fears and hopes they engender, the power of artificial intelligence (AI) and the capacities of robotics and genomics arouse both attraction and growing anxiety in humans. Some panicked at the idea of being dominated by machines made of carbon, tungsten, copper, and silicon, cold objects that would reduce us to the state of docile and stupid slaves. Others applauded, ready to sell their souls for a few clicks to the new digital happiness merchants. We are left speechless at the idea that we could give birth to beings shaped according to our own taste or acquire immortality that would mean the end of a humanity unable to mutate to adapt.

When I say augment it is not about improving the status of the sick or wounded for whom mechanical and digital assistance like connected prostheses allow them to regain their amputated capacities. Nor is it a question of refusing vaccination, which is not an augmentation but a simple activation of a natural immunological process, or of undergoing reconstructive or even esthetic surgery because we do not have surgery if we already consider ourselves as Venus or Apollo. It is the lack that leads to action. Another example: there is no augmentation in the use of medical therapies that combat impotence, but only a recovery of lost qualities. The most emblematic of the medical intrusions offered by digital techniques and AI are implants that reduce Parkinson tremors, digital aids for paralyzed people, or implantation of an artificial heart. Such aids have their constraints that are accepted as are the complications of conventional therapies provided they offer a greater advantage.

When it comes to healthy human beings it is perfectly lawful to help them accomplish tasks of strength thanks to exoskeletons, tools which do not violate the intimacy of the person, while ensuring them less painful activity. Other visual and hearing aids are multiplying leaving the individual completely free to use them for beneficial effects.

G. Vallancien (✉)
National Academy of Medicine, Washington, USA
e-mail: guy@vallancien.fr

© Springer Nature Switzerland AG 2020
B. Nordlinger et al. (eds.), *Healthcare and Artificial Intelligence*,
https://doi.org/10.1007/978-3-030-32161-1_33

On the other hand, augmenting memory or intelligence to "do more" through intrusive processes is a real problem, equal to that of facilitating drugs whose harmful effects are sometimes dramatic because of the addiction they cause. Too often, we play with words to leave an unhealthy blur about these differences that are the first conditions of an ethics of the human–machine relationship. In other words, this begs the question as to whether AI might be used to enslave us.

Is it logical to want to augment capacity in an artificial way when Lance Armstrong who cheated by taking drugs had to pay EUR5 million to settle a US federal complaint and suffer the cancellation of his seven victories at the Tour de France? Will we accept digital dopants when we refuse chemical doping?

Ray Kurzweil foresees the emergence in 2040 of such machines acquiring consciousness as if it were enough to add layers of computer chips on top of one another—roughly mimicking our brain function. Big deal! This scheme, because of its simplistic considerations, represents a box office hit. However, we must acknowledge the gap between the current capacities of instruments and the delirious promises made by their promoters. The very term "artificial intelligence" is inappropriate for several reasons!

It limits global intelligence, the exceptional capacity for adaptation and communication, to the sphere of gross calculation, ignoring what the senses bring to the brain. It therefore omits emotion, as well as all other forms of creative intelligence, whether manual, artistic, social, or amorous. Will the stonemason or reamer, violinist, drummer or poet, caregiver and childcare worker be classified in the category of simple process effectors, without creativity, madness or passion, without love, without laughter or tears?

To see or hear about the so-called artistic achievements of calculating machines allows us to measure the abyss that separates humans from computers. Toyota's violin robot delivers a sour sound, scraping its bow with a gesture offering no emotional resonance. The paintings created by Google form frescoes that are perfect for display in a hotel lobby—decorative at best. Such products have no history, no empathy; their productions are flat, empty as they are of meaning. Robots and AI tell us nothing. They act as gifted automatons that have never suffered—it is commonly believed you must have often cried to be able to create.

Human intelligence, slow and limited in the analysis of data, can become dazzling, capable of making immediate choices when encountering the unexpected and improbable, by bypassing all reasonable scenarios. It can anticipate, thwarting habits and standards like no other machine can, since it does not know the risk. Bringing together shared cognitive and emotional capacities whose substrate is biological. By constantly changing, mutating, and solicited by countless flows of information our global intelligence forms an architectural complex built on our genes, our individual being, and collective epigenetic variations resulting from our body sensations, our education, our climate, our food, social and cultural environments that modulate our behavior, our ways of thinking, and our beliefs. Wanting to compare a silicon chip with a neuron or a quantum computer with the human brain is as childish as comparing a lead soldier with a legionnaire in battle, or a mechanical automaton with a

2-year-old child. Computers are not smart. They classify a considerable accumulation of data to modulate the results statically.

In deep learning machines learn from their mistakes like us. But will they sacrifice themselves in the name of an ideal? Will we ever see a humanoid robot standing in front of army tanks in Tiananmen Square?

If you compare the most powerful calculator, which provides nearly 100 petaflops or 100 million billion operations per second, with what a 2-year-old child does the machine is ridiculously narrow-minded and linear. To recognize a cat or a dog requires millions of images viewed by computers, while a child after two or three tries understands immediately and is rarely mistaken. The first is ridiculous compared with the second.

Evaluating intelligence through tests quantifying intellectual quotient is a dramatically reducing way of assessing the value of human beings. What is the relationship between an IQ of 140 and self-sacrifice? What is the relationship between a standardized analysis test and the quality of a friendship, of sharing? Computers work fast, very fast, sometimes too fast, leading to aberrant decisions. They manipulate numbers to thousands of digits. Although their superiority in limited, bounded, and modelizable areas is undeniable, Alphago Zero would be totally lost if we added a line of squares to the Goban on which players challenge one another. It would stop, unable to invent a solution to a space of action that it ignores, because it has not been programmed—while a human being would immediately adapt to this new situation. Talking about AI is therefore a semantic usurpation, full of meaning because by using a word that covers extremely diverse concomitant thoughts and actions, we water down what makes us human with our creative follies, mixed in with lack and error. Intelligence is reduced to a processor and a memory without any other quality.

Human intelligence is multifaceted, not modelizable, because it is changing, constantly emerging during our conscious life. If the cerebral cortex works unceasingly, even during sleep phases, under the input of information from my inner environment and the world around me, without the body it would only be a pile of cells weighing 1300 g composed mainly of water and fat, nothing very original. It is the permanent relationship in proactive and retroactive loops between the body and the brain that creates the consciousness of being. Body and mind are consubstantial and inseparable, composed of the same molecules in an indescribable alchemy of sensations and reflections that form my person, unique, different from yours, the ultimate in creative biodiversity in perpetual renewal.

Some think that we will be able to analyze the modes of information within us by calculating their relevance, by copying them before redistributing them. We have no idea what is happening in our neurons and in our glial cells, their neighbors that we forget too often. We observe alpha, beta, gamma, and theta waves on the electroencephalogram, rudimentary signals of which we have limited understanding. The same frustration exhibits itself in our understanding of the excitement of the multiple brain areas that illuminate during a dynamic nuclear magnetic resonance (NMR) examination. Some neurological symptoms are linked to brain areas. We stop Parkinson tremors and restore memory to patients by exciting specific areas of the brain, bravo! But what exactly happens in the privacy of these billions of nerve cells, each linked to others by networks of thousands of connections. How is information transmitted by means of a subtle interplay between electrical waves and the flow of chemicals delivering a perfectly generated calibrated message? No one knows. The machines, on the other hand, operate in binary mode, 0 or 1, a thousand miles away from our biological plasticity. Will quantum computers raise the level of this triviality from all or nothing by refining their answers? Will they be able to manage the "a little," the "maybe," and the "why not"?

Sure that in the long run we will be able to understand and imitate the mechanisms that make us human, love and hate, laughter and tears, singing and dancing, some demiurges would like to improve us under the absurd pretext of not losing ground in the race for petaflops. Have a good trip to the land of fools! Will I be more attentive to others, will I have more capacity for empathy and love, stuffed with intracerebral chips sold by Neuralink, Elon Musk's firm? Any intrusion into my body as a healthy man by a connected tool that would give me greater cognitive abilities would be a rape of my very person. I would inevitably become the object of those who placed the chip in me, and I would also be at risk of being attacked by malicious hackers in jeans and Stan Smith sneakers living on the other side of the world to ransom me or make me their slave. Enhancing me as I am? The answer is no!

I want to remain free in myself with all my dreams, all my emotions, all my faults and limitations that make up my human wealth. To want to improve ourselves to be perfect is a chimera that would plunge us into eternal boredom. All of us "perfect" in the long term, all identical in single file since perfection is one. Hell, not that of the forked devil surrounded by flames, no, the real one, in the unbearable uniformity of the ideal being.

As a doctor, I will use all digital and genomic means to repair sick, injured, or disabled men, women, and children. However, I will never commit to increasing our capacities if diseases have not reduced them. Computers serve me every day as diagnostic or therapeutic decision support systems essential to improving patient care by reducing margins of error or as surgical robotics enabling actions at the very core of human anatomy. But the big juicy global market for augmentation is a perversion of humanity that I condemn. However, humans are what they are, capable of letting themselves be tempted. When they have created a monster from scratch, they may understand that nature cannot be played with with impunity. While we are the most accomplished living beings of evolution, we are not the masters.

To avoid such temptations let us organize a conference of parties (COP) on AI that will assess the expected benefits weighed against these risks. It would be France's honor to initiate this global awareness by moving away from the absurd cleavage between so-called bioconservatives and technoprogressists, old-fashioned denominations that lock each other in maximalist postures unworthy of humans and their values.

# Artificial Intelligence: A Vector for the Evolution of Health Professions and the Organization of Hospitals

Jean-Patrick Lajonchère

Today's health professions face major challenges that require assistance in terms of day-to-day practices, as well as improvements in collective modes of practice and management processes

In industrialized countries health security requires the right therapeutic attitude be guaranteed to patients. It is also necessary to be able to provide patients with evidence that they have received the proper implementation of medicine. To this end (particularly, in hospitals) quality processes are constantly being improved and increasingly monitored. At the same time, the acceleration and evaluation of research and research results makes it essential to maintain practitioner knowledge to enable the most suitable and up-to-date care.

All this impacts other health professions; medical progress needs support and the strengthening of existing procedures requires permanent adaptation and continuous staff training.

Patients' legitimate demands for quick access to care and shorter hospital stays require an organization that is constantly being optimized to meet such demands.

Moreover, the need for networking with health professionals who support patients outside hospital therefore affects all staff. Such optimization must also facilitate financial sustainability in healthcare systems; the reduction of additional costs is particularly linked to a required improvement in coordination between professionals.

All healthcare professions therefore need to adapt to meet future challenges. Complexity is at the heart of these challenges incorporating quantity of data, multiplicity of situations, technicality of care, diversity of support required, patient requirements, real-time expertise, etc.

Human intelligence has reached the point where the continued development of expertise and management requires technological assistance; over the past few

J.-P. Lajonchère (✉)
Paris Saint-Joseph Hospital Group, chargé de mission to the Minister of Europe and Foreign Affairs for Export Health Support, Paris, France
e-mail: JPLajonchere@hpsj.fr

© Springer Nature Switzerland AG 2020
B. Nordlinger et al. (eds.), *Healthcare and Artificial Intelligence*,
https://doi.org/10.1007/978-3-030-32161-1_34

decades computers and software have increasingly advanced expertise and management systems. However, quantity of data and the speed of responses required to manage the multiplicity of situations require decision support tools that are more adaptable and powerful than those available today. Artificial intelligence should provide a solution thanks to powerful computers and software running complex algorithms. The ability of this technology to quickly analyze large amounts of data is currently being used for applied research. Such technology will strengthen the power and scalability of expertise, systematization of data processing, the use of real-time knowledge banks, the analysis of images and texts, etc. It is not a question of replacing human intervention—a fear that is omnipresent—but of complementing it, guiding it, rationalizing it, and monitoring it. Since the earliest of times, humans and the media have used instruments to help with and extend their reach. Historically, innovation has always raised questions. Artificial intelligence is no exception. However, in medicine the link between patients and healthcare professionals remains at the heart of medical practice. There is nothing to suggest that such relationships between patients and professionals would be adversely affected by the use of decision support tools.

Contributions from artificial intelligence are multifaceted and have consequences for both organizations and professions. Many applications are already under development.

## For Hospitals

The use of artificial intelligence can be used to simplify issues such as the complexity of treatment for chronic diseases associated with old age and the optimization of unprogrammed management.

In emergency room admissions artificial intelligence can be used to improve the likelihood that patients receive the right clinical assessment and therefore are provided with optimal treatments. Such assessments need to be based on real-time analysis of the current situation of a patient alongside their medical and social history and the use of data available through shared medical records and other data collected under similar conditions. The creation of analytical tools based on good practice will help make clinical decisions more reliable.

Early real-time identification of patients potentially carrying multidrug-resistant bacteria is currently being developed. This will improve risk management within hospitals. Such systems involve the implementation of preventive procedures for surveillance, hygiene, and septic isolation reinforcing the personalized control of infection risk.

Being able to predict which patients are at risk of deteriorating is of critical importance; real-time analysis of parameters and data from patients will make this a reality. Subsequently, surveillance and care can be systematized. This can at the level of each healthcare facility either prevent resuscitation visits or anticipate and manage them. In both cases continuous data analysis—something doctors cannot do—using artificial intelligence will lead to considerable improvement in the personalization of care.

These examples show that hospitals will very soon be at the center of so-called "P4" medicine (i.e., medicine that is predictive, preventive, personalized, and participatory). How biology (the study of living things) integrating the analysis of environmental and societal factors evolves will concern research units and collaborative platforms. Such analyses should be based on getting biologists, clinicians, sociologists, and bioinformaticians to associate in the application of research results. Once again the use of artificial intelligence will be able to guide and pool expertise.

The contribution made by artificial intelligence will only be really effective in combination with data exchange technologies and the most advanced office automation tools such as voice recognition. Thus, a patient's medical, pharmaceutical, and medicosocial file would need to be completed in real time—the only way to make such an analysis effective.

It is therefore necessary for hospitals to undertake and complete a transformation to digital to be able to enter into processes like data exchange. Current trends in collaborative functioning within health regions should help to accelerate this process.

Of course, hospitals are also institutions that must enable medicine to be practiced and care to be coordinated. As such, hospitals are probably the most complex societal organizations in the industrial and service sectors combining security constraints (e.g., in operating theaters) and coordination between complementary processes, each with their own constraints (hospitalization, consultation, and imaging), supported by healthcare professionals as well as logisticians, technicians, and administrative staff.

Although optimizing such work processes has partly been achieved and hospitalization time is shortening, it is up to each individual organization to adapt such processes. A large university hospital must schedule more than 100 surgical procedures and around 300 scans and magnetic resonance imaging (MRI) scans daily. The management of "hospital flows" in terms of imaging or procedures in operating theaters should make it possible to optimize resources and secure all routes. This needs to be based on more efficient systems than we have today so that caregivers remain focused on the act of care, free from the worries of daily organization. The scheduling and coordination of more than one examination for a patient can be improved because the current complexity of implementation often constitutes a limit to waiting times for such technical platforms. Delays in obtaining appointments and waiting times for tests or consultations affect the management of patients and can lead to a loss of confidence in hospitals. A real-time analysis of activity will make it possible to adapt the workforce at appropriate times.

Safety in operating theaters can be improved by the actions of permanent analysis medical teams providing a means of anticipating and preventing errors.

The entire drug supply process can be made safer by the use of real-time prescribing and analyzing prescriptions in terms of previous treatments and iatrogenic data.

Hopefully, in the near future hospitals will benefit from artificial intelligence providing organizational support.

# For Professionals

As far as professionals are concerned it can be estimated that they will be supported by artificial intelligence on two levels: expertise in fields using imagery and diagnostic assistance based on database studies.

## Doctors

Three fields of application and assistance for doctors are foreseeable:

1. Strengthening the capacity for establishing the prognosis, therapy, and follow-up to cancer treatments.
    Specifically, this will be achieved by improving activities that are currently limited by the analytical capacity of human beings.
2. Diagnostic assistance with imaging, dermatology, ophthalmology, cardiology, and pathological anatomy (specifically, by facilitating the analysis of ever-increasing numbers of images). Artificial intelligence, a tool derived from current computer-aided diagnostics, provides great processing power and will one day be able to complete the analysis of images in conjunction with clinical data. Research is currently under development with products coming onto the market (breast, cardiac MRI, etc.).
3. Improving diagnostic reliability the evolution of which may take time. The aim is to reliably extract unstructured data elements and to build, on the basis of research, analytical models that achieve performances equal to or better than those achieved by human beings.

## Researchers

First and foremost, the debate on making clinical trial data available must be resolved. The objective here is to enable this. This is already the case for data from European marketing authorization dossiers. Subsequent to access to such data researchers will be able to analyze, for example, the risks and benefits of drugs.

Such data analysis will accelerate the induction of new cohorts into the field of artificial intelligence; mathematicians will continue to be attracted by the field and bioinformaticians will be omnipresent.

Supporting the inclusion of patients in research protocols is a routine application that will benefit clinician researchers. Watson for Clinical Trials Matching identifies patients who might benefit from research protocols being implemented in hospitals. The company's figures indicate a 78% reduction in the medical time required for patient inclusion into such schemes.

## *Other Trades*

Nurses or medical assistants will be guided in their routines such as connecting systems, prescription reminders, and real-time deviation measurement. Radiologists will benefit through simplification driven by adaptive devices that reduces the complexity of imaging systems and their means of interfacing with management software.

Porters will have their journeys optimized reducing distances walked and thereby waiting times.

Logisticians will therefore have at their disposal expert systems for organizing operating theaters, laboratories, imaging facilities, and emergency departments. Such systems are already used in the hotel or air transport industries benefiting management and reducing errors and uncertainty.

Pharmacists will benefit through the automatic application of drug contraindication verification, with the search for iatrogeny becoming systematic, including treatments available to patients outside hospitals.

Administrative and management professions will also benefit from such analyses enabling the improvement of a hospital's economic performance without degrading its quality of care. In fact, such an approach to the optimization of resources, and thereby improved efficiency, greatly benefits the service provided. The example of medical secretaries is illustrative on this point. The transition to all-digital patient records achieved through the use of voice recognition reduces the need for secretaries to type letters to patients. Rather than using this technology to eliminate employment in this sector, it would be more appropriate to develop the role of medical secretaries in terms of strengthening their presence to patients using them to reassure and provide guidance to patients. It is anticipated that similar examples will become apparent as a consequence of artificial intelligence. This becomes an opportunity for healthcare providers to offer greater levels of support to patients.

Artificial intelligence will in fact raise professional standards providing assistance based on comprehensive, rationalized assumptions and data.

## Patients and Public Health

Big Data can feed on information transmitted from connected objects. They will inexorably continue to spread. It is estimated that 161 million health devices will be connected worldwide in 2020. Taking better charge of your health, guided by personalized expertise, is one of the "big dreams" of visionaries of Big Data and artificial intelligence. Although currently this ambitious objective is far from being achieved, the provision of more reliable and targeted data certainly represents a potential source of greater accountability for everyone. Patient associations will need to be included in such a system to better fulfill their role as upstream advisors. Based on a better knowledge of interactions, prediction and therefore prevention will better involve patients, allowing them the means to influence treatments through appropriate perspectives on their own health.

Calculation of the differences in actual or estimated coverage can benefit from the support of artificial intelligence. The aim is to analyze on a broader basis than present the performance of health systems across all professions and hospitals.

Some 5% of patients in public health in the United States account for 50% of healthcare spending. This is likely similar in France. Identification of such patients should make it possible to set up appropriate care leading to an improvement in their state of health and therefore potential community savings. Thus, the "mechanism of the future" will be able to integrate, beyond pathology, all the biological, behavioral, and environmental variables enabling a diagnosis to be made and an appropriate treatment to be proposed.

The management of hospital emergency services could benefit from the analysis of information from pharmacies on increased drug purchases—considered precursors to epidemics.

## Conclusion: What Will Be the Likely Impact on Medical Professions and the Training of Professionals?

It is unlikely that the introduction of artificial intelligence in hospitals and more generally in the health sector as a whole will lead to job savings. As Cédric Villani's report titled "Defence in the Age of AI" indicates, few hospital or health tasks are self-contained. Indeed, the need for social interaction in the field of care is omnipresent, and the need to be able to solve difficulties in each profession independently is permanent. The human being remains at the center of the system.

The main challenge is to promote complementary action between health professionals and technology. Expertise will have to adapt, and initial and continuing training will need to prepare professionals for this new expertise.

We will need more engineers, statisticians, and data scientists. However, health professionals will need to maintain a continuous link with patients while strengthening their presence in all these additional technological processes.

By strengthening expertise we must strive to strengthen human beings: "high tech, high touch." Health professionals will need to learn to use artificial intelligence and be aware of its limitations and conditions of use. Social networks can pose a risk to the preservation of confidentiality. Similarly, the lack of objectivity in the use of artificial intelligence, or its withdrawal into applications apparently distanced from patients, can represent a real issue.

More training in social sciences must be integrated into health professions to support the technological strengthening required.

Some concerns are:

1. Will current trades disappear? In health fields, no. Many will however have to adapt and evolve toward more expertise provided by technology.

2. Will doctors lose their free will? No. They will have a permanent, rational, literary, and knowledgeable assistant to guide their expertise, but the final decision will remain with them.
3. Will medicine become dehumanized with the addition of artificial intelligence? No. However, it will be necessary to strengthen the training given in social science courses.

To this end medical schools and medical professions will have to adapt and continuously integrate new technologies incorporating their consequences and limitations into teaching. As access to knowledge becomes easier it will be necessary, even more so than today, to learn how to learn. Flexibility of programs making them continuously adaptable should become the rule. Associations with engineering schools and faculties of human sciences will be essential.

Artificial intelligence holds great promise through its ability to strengthen expertise, its potential for research dynamics, and its capability to optimize logistics and organizational systems. It is also a source of potential risk (particularly, in terms of confidentiality). Preparing all health professionals for the future means enabling them to safely integrate this potentially powerful tool, which should make it possible to push the boundaries of medicine and therefore meet the goal of improving human health.

Printed in the United States
by Baker & Taylor Publisher Services